Praise for *The Martial Arts of Vietnam* ..

We are truly indebted to Master Augustus Roe (Võ sư Quảng Thừa, 廣乘武師) for writing this book. In it, he not only shares the unique experiences he gained as he sought out martial artists throughout Vietnam, but also opens up for us their traditions, cultural practices, histories, stories, philosophies, and beliefs. Moreover, Augustus Roe's insights into Vietnam's ethnic, regional, and cultural diversity allow us to more fully appreciate the martial arts culture of Vietnam's lands and peoples.

> —Venerable Quang Huyen, Buddhist monk of Xá Lợi Pagoda, PhD in Vietnamese literature and culture, author of Dharma Mountain Buddhism & Martial Yoga

This is a very important piece of work written by someone who knows what they are writing about. It is a detailed exploration of the various Vietnamese martial arts, both foreign and indigenous, that fills a gap in the available research on combative systems. Both informative and interesting, this book will surely stimulate further research and debate on the subject. A ten out of ten!

> —Jamie Lee Baron Hanshi, president of the Institute of Martial Arts and Sciences, Accrington, Lancashire, United Kingdom

Augustus John Roe has done a fine job of helping us understand Vietnamese martial arts by first researching the history of Vietnam. For example, the historical relationship between China and Vietnam explains Chinese influence in Vietnamese martial arts. And knowing that three hundred thousand South Vietnamese troops fought alongside the Americans during the Vietnam conflict explains how taekwondo arrived in Vietnam. Of particular interest to me was the section on traditional Vietnamese wrestling, about which very little has been previously written. This book represents an amazing amount of research and is a valuable contribution to the body of knowledge in the field of martial arts, history, and culture.

> —Dr. Antonio Graceffo, PhD from Shanghai University of Sport Wushu Department, author, black belt in Cambodian martial arts

THE MARTIAL ARTS OF VIETNAM

THE MARTIAL ARTS OF VIETNAM
AN OVERVIEW OF HISTORY AND STYLES

- AUGUSTUS JOHN ROE -

YMAA Publication Center
Wolfeboro, NH USA

YMAA Publication Center, Inc.
PO Box 480
Wolfeboro, New Hampshire 03894
1-800-669-8892 • info@ymaa.com • www.ymaa.com

ISBN: 9781594397974 (print) • ISBN: 9781594397981 (ebook)

Publisher's Cataloging in Publication

Names: Roe, Augustus John, 1988- author.

Title: The martial arts of Vietnam : an overview of history and styles / Augustus John Roe.

Description: Wolfeboro, NH USA : YMAA Publication Center, [2020] | Includes bibliographical references.

Identifiers: ISBN: 9781594397974 (print) | 9781594397981 (Ebook) | LCCN: 2020939624

Subjects: LCSH: Martial arts--Vietnam. | Martial arts--Vietnam--History. | Martial arts--Vietnam --Pictorial works. | Martial arts schools--Vietnam--Directories. | BISAC: SPORTS & RECREATION / Martial Arts. | HEALTH & FITNESS / Tai Chi. | HISTORY / Asia / Southeast Asia.

Classification: LCC: GV1100.73 .R64 2020 | DDC: 796.8/0957--dc23

- DEDICATED TO ISSY & ALYSSA -

CONTENTS

Notes on the Writing of Non-English Words

The Vietnamese language is generally written using characters of the Latin alphabet with diacritical markings indicating tonal inflections and various vowel sounds. However, with the exception of italicized words and occasional logographs that are included alongside English translations, throughout the majority of this book the Romanized spellings of Vietnamese words are used. Therefore, words such as *Hà Nội* and *Hồ Chí Minh* have been transcribed as Hanoi and Ho Chi Minh, respectively. All words written using the Vietnamese script have been included in the glossary for reference, as have specific martial arts terms written as Romanizations of other languages, such as *Qi, Qigong, Chi Sao* and *Gi.* Furthermore, the terms *Master, Grandmaster* and *Patriarch Master* have been used to refer to an instructor who has achieved mastery of an art form or a rank that designates them the title, the current or former head of a school or system and the deceased founder of an individual school or style, respectively.

INTRODUCTION

Since the beginning of recorded history, violence has been an inescapable part of human nature. In attempts to organize this violence, codified systems of combat that "blend the physical components with strategy, philosophy, tradition, or other features"[1] have developed. In this book, these modern expressions of our violent nature, known as "martial arts" will be examined in the context of the lands we now call Vietnam.

This book will focus upon the forms of "cold" (i.e. non-firearm-based) martial arts that exist in various forms today. As a study of embodied culture, we will consider the ways in which the people of Vietnam find meaning in the historical narratives and modern practices of martial arts. As we shall see, the martial culture and history of the region is exciting and diverse, with everything from warring swordswomen and tiger-felling martial monks to pirates and wrestlers-turned-kings.

Upon first arriving In Vietnam more than a decade ago, I was astounded by both the range of martial arts on display and the pride the Vietnamese people took in their practices. In contrast, it was a shock to learn that the martial arts of a nation with such a rich culture of combat were so little known to the outside world.

After several years studying and then teaching Vietnamese martial arts, I found myself needing to describe these systems and as a result, wanting to learn more about them myself. I then traveled to all corners of the nation seeking out knowledge and skills. I found myself plunged into countryside wrestling contests, being thrown across dusty temple courtyards by the descendants of famous warrior clans and navigating the floodplains of the Mekong delta in search of legendary martial arts masters.

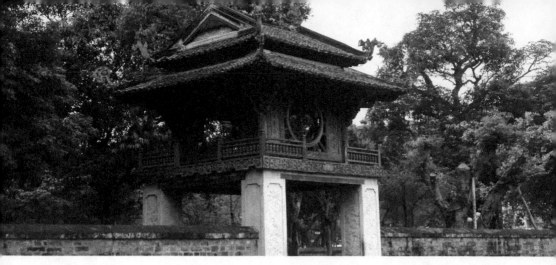

*The main gate of Van Mieu Quoc Tu Giam in Hanoi,
which hosted the royal court's examinations from the tenth century*

This book emerges out of my ruminations and my attempt to share these traditions and the knowledge I have accumulated with audiences beyond Vietnam.

Although the present-day incarnation of the country was not even formed until the late eighteenth century, the coming text considers modern Vietnamese martial arts, therefore we will include all of those that have developed within Vietnam's current borders. This covers a huge range of unique and interesting practices, that play important social, cultural, spiritual and physical roles in the nation. We intend to introduce some of these martial arts schools and systems in regards to their physical practices, how they fit into both the local and global martial arts scene, and finally, what they reveal about Vietnam's exciting and turbulent martial history.

Although there are a number of thematic ways to consider Vietnamese martial arts (for example in relation to religion or ethnicity), within this book they have been categorized by geographical location. The main reasons for this being the historical, cultural and geographical differences between the north, central and southern regions of Vietnam. Within these areas, inhabitants see themselves as culturally (and in some cases ethnically) distinct from their countrymen. As a result of these factors, localized cultures have developed, with each group holding their own values, traditions and understanding of what martial arts mean to them.

It should be highlighted to the reader that, although this book contains information on a variety of Vietnamese martial arts, it is by no means a comprehensive encyclopedia of schools and styles and should be used only as an introduction to the nation's martial arts systems and cultures. Furthermore, this book describes only those that have large followings in Vietnam. Although hundreds of Vietnamese-lineage styles exist in other parts of the world, due to cultural differences, they have not been included here.

It should also be noted that, like all modern-day countries, the cultures and identities of the people living in Vietnam are varied and ever-changing. As a result, any references in this book to specific areas of land, ethnicities or races are purely descriptive terms and, in some cases, may not be fully representative of the current situation.

Finally, it must be made clear that this is not an instructional document and all martial arts training must only be undertaken with the guidance of a professional and qualified instructor.

OVERVIEW

OF

VIETNAM

&

KEY

MARTIAL

HISTORY

TIMELINE OF VIETNAM

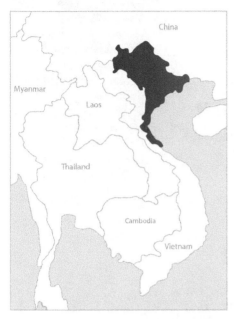

2879–258 BCE		Hồng Bàng Dynasty
2879–1913 BCE		Early Hồng Bàng
1912–1055 BCE		Mid-Hồng Bàng
1054–258 BCE		Late Hồng Bàng
257–179 BCE		Thục Dynasty
207–111 BCE		Triệu Dynasty

■ The Nam Viet (Nan Yue) Kingdom - Circa 300 BCE
☐ Modern Southeast Asia

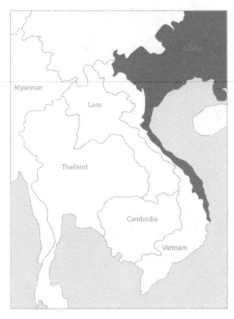

111 BC–40 CE		1st Chinese Era
40–43 CE		Trưng Sisters Uprising
43–544 CE		2nd Chinese Era
544–602 CE		Early Lý Dynasty
602–938 CE		3rd Chinese Era

■ The Nam Viet Kingdom after takeover from the
Han Chinese - Circa 111 BCE
☐ Modern Southeast Asia

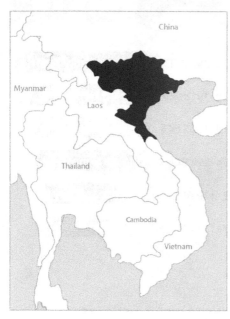

939–967	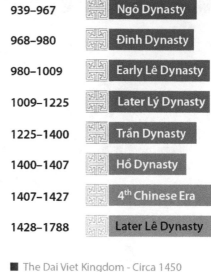	Ngô Dynasty
968–980		Đinh Dynasty
980–1009		Early Lê Dynasty
1009–1225		Later Lý Dynasty
1225–1400		Trần Dynasty
1400–1407		Hồ Dynasty
1407–1427		4th Chinese Era
1428–1788		Later Lê Dynasty

■ The Dai Viet Kingdom - Circa 1450
☐ Modern Southeast Asia

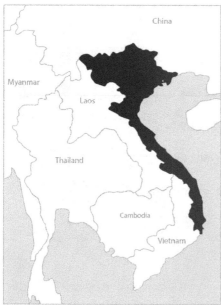

1527–1592	Mạc Dynasty
1545–1787	Trịnh Lords
1558–1777	Nguyễn Lords
1778–1802	Tây Sơn Dynasty
1802–1945	Nguyễn Dynasty

■ The Dai Viet Kingodm - Circa 1780
☐ Modern Southeast Asia

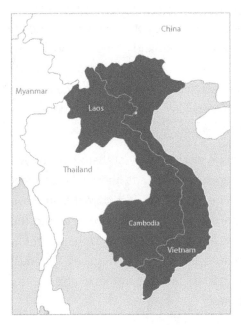

1858–1945   **French Imperialism**

1945–1954   **Post-Colonial Vietnam**

◼ French Indochina - Circa 1930
▢ Modern Southeast Asia

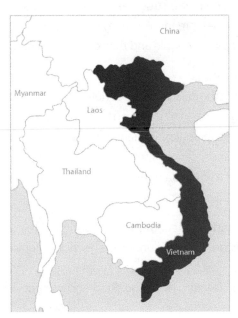

1954 – 1975   **North/South Vietnam**

From 1975   **Socialist Republic**

◼ Modern-Day Vietnam
▢ Modern Southeast Asia

Vietnam has a land mass close to 332,000 square kilometers, it borders China to the north, mainland Southeast Asia to the west and has hundreds of kilometers of coastline. As a result, the region has long been seen as a strategically and economically valuable resource. The modern incarnation of Vietnam was first amalgamated by military expansion southwards throughout the seventeenth century, giving the country its distinct "S" shape. Meanwhile, the northern borders have had very little modification since the withdrawal of the Song Dynasty in 1070.[2]

Vietnam has a total of fifty-four ethnic groups. Although many of them have played important roles in the development of the region's martial arts, those who consider themselves to be ethnically Vietnamese (referred to as the **Việt** or **Viet-Kinh**) have undeniably had the most impact on modern practices. The Viet have inhabited the Red River Delta region for centuries and while the Chinese empire to the north has had a profound influence upon the local culture and its martial practices, a gradual southwards expansion of the Viet into unknown lands further "transformed this country into a mosaic of peoples, languages, and cultures."[3]

Within this diverse and often dangerous region, countless struggles for dominance, land and survival took place. This in turn led to the development of an array of unique martial arts practices that have been shaped not just by the people and their cultures, but also by the very landscape itself.

Geographical factors have had huge impacts on the development of Vietnamese martial arts. Aspects such as climate and agricultural accessibility shaped numerous military campaigns, while more specific examples of geographical influences can be observed within martial practices themselves. For instance, certain methods of high stepping appear in some arts that may be more suited to mountainous terrains, while styles of gripping and locking that are adapted for extremely humid climates appear in others.

In modern times, the general population consider their country as consisting of three key areas (this is likely due in part to a historical divide under the French colonial administration). Each of these three regions can be considered as cultural spheres, with observable differences in ethnicity, attitudes, religion, language, food and of course, martial arts.

- The Northern Region (formerly referred to as Tonkin by the French) is inhabited primarily by the Viet people surrounding the capital city of Hanoi and the Red River Delta. While the Tay, Tai, Muong, Nung and Hmong ethnic groups reside in the surrounding highlands to the north and west. While the Red River Delta has historically served as a crossroad for both migrations and trade with China, the Chinese influence, particularly on the northern Vietnamese culture (and therefore its martial arts) has been profound. The north of the country predominantly cites no specific religious affiliations, but widely follows a number of Daoist and Folk religious practices alongside Buddhism.

- The Central Region (formerly Annam), consists of beautiful coastal lowlands to the east which are inhabited by a mixture of the Viet, Hoa (Chinese) and Cham (an ethnic group well known for their historical warrior culture).[4] To the west sit highlands that are inhabited by the Viet and numerous other peoples such as the Bahnar, Ede, Jarai and others. Catholicism, Hinduism, Islam and a number of tribal religions are common among the citizens of the central provinces.

- The Southern Region (formerly Cochinchina), consists of lowlands surrounding the metropolis of Ho Chi Minh City and the Mekong Delta as well as highlands to the north and west. Major ethnicities include the Viet, Hoa, Cham, Khmer and other smaller ethnic groups, all of which have held power in the region over the centuries and have contributed to the development of the Southern Vietnamese martial arts. A wider range of religious practices can typically be observed in the southern provinces compared to the north of the country. These include Mahayana, Theravada and Hoa Hao Buddhism as well as Catholicism and Caodaism.

The modern nation consists of fifty-eight individual provinces—areas that have their own administration but are governed by central leadership. The Viet people account for the vast majority of the population, however the Tai, Cham, Khmer, Bahnar and Jarai were all once physically and culturally dominant powers in the region.[5] The Cham and Khmer in particular, controlled vast swathes of Southeast Asia and their influences can still be observed in the diversity of Vietnam's martial practices today.

Furthermore, the population of modern Vietnam is extremely young (with almost half of the approximate ninety-four million residents aged below twenty-nine).[6] This factor coupled with an increasing national wage and social welfare system has lent itself well to the ongoing development and practice of martial arts by the current generation.

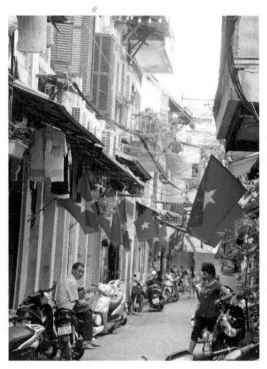

Vietnamese flags line many of the streets in Hanoi

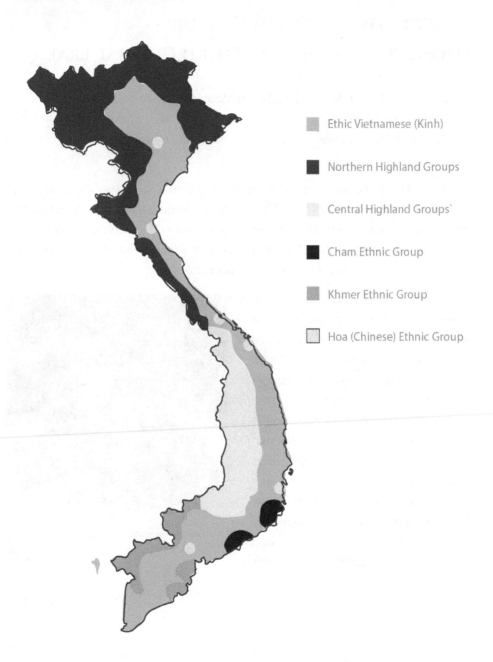

Ethic Vietnamese (Kinh)

Northern Highland Groups

Central Highland Groups`

Cham Ethnic Group

Khmer Ethnic Group

Hoa (Chinese) Ethnic Group

Key Martial History

Early History—Tenth Century (Hong Bang Dynasty—Third Chinese Era)

Around 2000 BCE, the **Đông Sơn** (literally **East Mountain**) culture developed into a thriving civilization around the Red River Delta. Weapons such as swords, spears, daggers and axes and intricately decorated war drums which depict battle scenes, have been discovered in the region.

Between 111 BCE and 938 CE, the Red River Delta region fluctuated between rulers from the northern region (of what is now China) and local leaders. **Nan Yue** (or **Nam Việt**) as it was known at the time, was desirable due to its agricultural opportunities (in contrast to the mountainous highlands to the north), strategic military placement and as an access route to trading across the south seas and Indian Ocean.[7]

During the first millennium, it is considered that the occupants of the Red River Delta lived in "relative peace and security as residents of the Sinitic empire."[8] Despite this, a number of stories detailing uprisings against the ruling dynasties have found their way into the modern Vietnamese canon, such as that of the Two Trung Sisters (*Hai Bà Trưng*), from today's Ba Vi area of northern Vietnam. The pair are said to have been fearsome warriors, who overthrew the ruling Han Dynasty and briefly seized control, before succumbing to Han forces two years later.

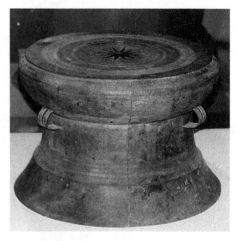

A Dong Son drum on display in the Vietnamese Museum of Vietnamese history

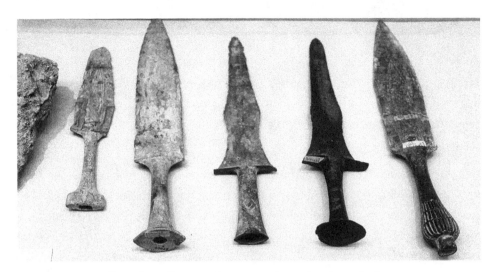

Hong Bang Dynasty daggers and spearheads on display in the Museum of Vietnamese history

TENTH—SIXTEENTH CENTURY
(NGO DYNASTY—MAC DYNASTY)

In 1009 a Buddhist martial artist named Ly Cong Uan (crowned Ly Thai To) rose to power, founding the Ly Dynasty which lasted until 1225. The emperor was raised in a Buddhist temple and "had a reputation for both erudition and martial prowess."[9]

During the Ly Dynasty, the Buddhist clergy were closely associated with the Emperor's household. Buddhism was elevated to an official religion and prospered alongside various other Daoist, spiritual and other shamanistic practices. It is also claimed that in this period, the Buddhist clergy openly trained in martial arts and competed in festival tournaments that featured wrestling, boxing and empty-handed contests.[10]

The Ly Dynasty began a campaign of **Nam Tiến** (literally translated as **Marching South**) and gradually expanded their territory through fierce battles with the southern Khmer and Champa empires. The Cham were a historically renowned warrior culture, who regularly "fought each other and neither had any qualms about attacking the nascent **Đại Việt** state in the north to expand their own empires."[11] Coincidentally, the former Cham capital city **Indrapura**, is located in modern-day Quy Nhon, Binh Dinh Province, a region which in recent years has become considered by many to be "the cradle of Vietnamese martial arts." [12]

In 1253, the Tran Dynasty established one of the first formal martial arts training institutions in the capital (then known as *Thăng Long*). At that time, these schools were primarily for high-ranking military officers and relatives of the royal family, rather than the general public. [13]

In 1257, 1284 and 1287 the Mongol armies attempted invasions of the region then known as *Đại Việt* and were subsequently repelled. These victories are famed for the use of guerrilla tactics, led by General Tran Hung Dao. An example of this was baiting the Mongol army to sail down the Bach Dang River during low tide and lining the riverbed with iron-tipped stakes.

Mac Dang Dung, a warrior-official who had effectively controlled the country for over a decade, seized the throne in 1527. Mac Dang Dung was known as a skilled wrestler, renowned for his size, strength and accomplished military record. Some sources state that despite his position, he championed martial arts among his people and would often compete with civilian masters inside the Imperial Court, accepting those that bettered him into official positions. [11]

SEVENTEENTH CENTURY—EIGHTEENTH CENTURY (NGUYEN & TRINH LORDS—TAY SON DYNASTY)

In the early seventeenth century, following a number of violent disputes between provincial rulers, Nguyen Hoang (the figurehead of a military household from Thanh Hoa) fled the north and ventured south in an attempt to establish his own domain. Nguyen Hoang, his son Nguyen Phuc Nguyen and other members of their household began building a new state, developing military settlements across the coast and erecting Buddhist pagodas. The Nguyen family are said to have recruited numerous warriors and martial arts experts from the north to strengthen their new land and military. [15]

Under Nguyen Hoang and his successors, a number of the armed and unarmed martial arts practices were recorded by family clans in central Vietnam; most famously the

Truong Clan who stemmed from Thanh Hoa Province and moved south into Binh Dinh Province as vassals of the Nguyen. Their descendant, Truong Duc Giai, is credited with compiling a book that details fifteen forms of his family's martial arts styles. While a later descendant, Truong Van Hien, is said to have taught martial arts to the three warrior brothers of the Tay Son Rebellion. Many of these original documents survive today and are featured as the core practices of a family of martial arts referred to as *Võ Cổ Truyền* (literally *Traditional Vietnamese Martial Arts*).[16][17]

In 1721, the first public martial arts school was established in Thang Long (modern-day Hanoi) by King Le Du Tong.[18]

From the seventeenth century onwards, increasing numbers of Viet and ethnic Chinese (Hoa) immigrants settled the Mekong Delta region. This included several thousand former followers of the Chinese Ming Dynasty and numerous Viet martial arts experts and soldiers who had followed the Nguyen south.[19]

Cross cohabitation between Viet settlers and ethnic minority groups during the seventeenth and eighteenth centuries is likely to have led to further adaptations in the Southern Vietnamese martial arts. Around this time, many of the Viet settlers also relied on Buddhist sorcery and magic to protect themselves from danger. These superstitions were amplified by the harsh and mysterious environment of the south[20] and many such practices were further imbued into and practiced in conjunction with local martial arts.

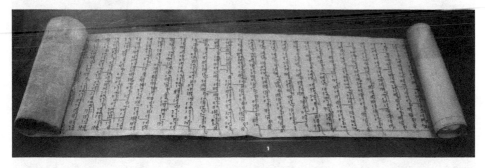

An eighteenth century Cham-Muslim Koran

Continued warfare and allegiances (through diplomacy and marriage) took place with the Khmer throughout the seventeenth and eighteenth centuries. During this period, the southwestern provinces of the Khmer Kingdom, including the city of **Prey Nokor** (modern-day Ho Chi Minh City) were gradually lost to the Viet. Although the Khmer have a long legacy as warriors (thousands of examples of artwork depicting martial arts practices can be observed in the ancient Khmer capital of **Angkor Wat**), a mixture of political and economic problems, military campaigns from the north and civil war had weakened the once dominant empire, allowing the Viet to deepen their grasp of the region.[21]

From 1771, the Tay Son Rebellion grew in the central province of Binh Dinh, led by three brothers (Nguyen Nhac, Nguyen Hue and Nguyen Lu). All of the Tay Son brothers were martial arts experts trained under various Chinese and Viet masters, most notably Truong Van Hien.[22] In 1773, the oldest brother (Nguyen Nhac) seized the former Cham capital city of Quy Nhon, Binh Dinh Province.

In a bid to consolidate their power, the Tay Son formed alliances with marginalized groups such as the ethnic highlanders, Khmer, Chinese, Cham and Viet Christians. All of the above are considered to have significantly impacted the rebellion, however none more dramatically than the vagabonds, bandits, and pirates recruited by the Tay Son, with Nguyen Hue even becoming known as "the rebel protector of pirates."[23]

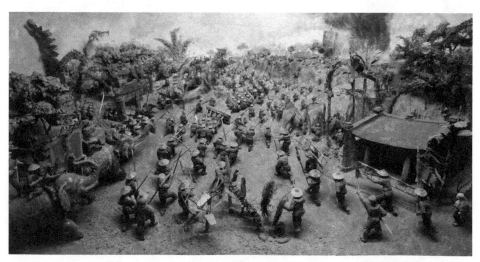

A scene depicting the battle of Ngoc Hoi—a key victory for the Tay Son Rebellion

Bui Thi Xuan was a general of the Tay Son Rebellion and expert of local (Binh Dinh) martial arts who trained under Master Ngo Manh, a former general of the Nguyen Dynasty.[24] Bui Thi Xuan allegedly "distinguished herself as a fierce commander of several thousand troops"[25] while she and her husband Tran Quang Dieu, led Tay Son fighters to victory in battles against the Siamese (modern-day Thai) and against Viet forces in Quy Nhon and Nghe An. In modern times, Bui Thi Xuan is still revered for her successes leading female squadrons and her expertise in swordsmanship.[26] She is credited with developing a form of dual-sword wielding known as **Song Phượng Kiếm** (*Phoenix Double-swords*) which is still widely practiced within Binh Dinh region martial arts systems.

In 1777 the Tay Son killed the Nguyen monarch and much of the Royal Family in the Saigon area. Five years later, they massacred some 10,000 Chinese Nguyen supporters. Finally, in 1786, the warrior-general Nguyen Hue stormed the nation's capital, leading 100,000 men and 100 elephants.[27] He took the throne of the first modern incarnation of the country, while his two brothers governed the central and southern regions. Nguyen Hue declared himself Emperor, taking on the name Quang Trung.

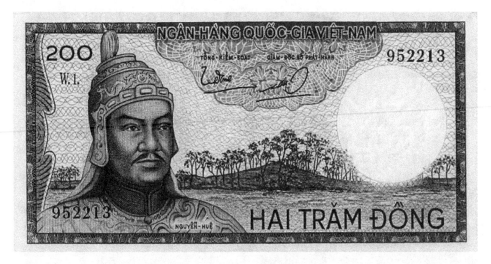

Fig. 1. A two hundred Dong note featuring the image of Quang Trung

Eighteenth—Nineteenth century
(Nguyen Dynasty—French Imperialism)

On the heels of the short-lived Tay Son Dynasty which fell after Quang Trung's death in 1802, the Nguyen Dynasty returned to power. Emperor Minh Manh reinstituted official martial arts examinations for both military and civilian practitioners. At the Nguyen Court in the Dynasty's new capital of Hue, ranks and degrees were awarded in both martial arts and military tactics; a total of 3,983 candidates passed martial examinations between 1802 and 1884.[28]

Throughout the eighteenth and nineteenth century, several major schools of Chinese martial arts such as Hung Gar, Bak Mei Pei and Wing Chun were recorded as popular practices in the Cholon market district of Saigon (now Ho Chi Minh City).[29]

The French invaded Vietnam in 1858 and managed to maintain control over the country (with nominal Nguyen Dynasty rule) until the middle of World War One. Under the French, the Vietnamese people faced economic and religious repression, while martial arts practices were also prohibited.[30] Although the French had a significant impact on modern Vietnamese culture, it is considered that such prohibition actually had the opposite of its intended effect, strengthening the practices of Buddhism and other related traditions—such as martial arts—by forcing them to develop new networks underground.[31]

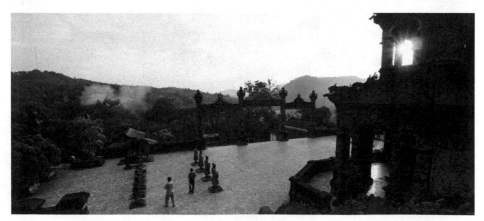

The Mausoleum of Nguyen Dynasty Kings on the outskirts of Hue City

During the late nineteenth and early twentieth centuries, there were numerous uprisings and revolts in the Seven Mountains region of Southwest Vietnam. An example of which is that orchestrated by the former soldier and martial arts expert, Tran Van Thanh of the *Bửu Sơn Kỳ Hương* Sect. Thanh led twelve hundred Khmer and Viet fighters in battles against the oppressive French regime in the 1860s.[32]

During the early twentieth century, the French recruited numerous soldiers from the central highlands and trained them as fighters (primarily from the Bahnar, Jarai and Rhade groups). Within this period, the military ethnographer Captain Maurice widely acknowledged both the spirit and skills of the recruits in conflict stating, "Today the warrior instincts of the (Rhade) tribe bloom within our *Batallions Montagnards (mountaineer battalions)*."[33]

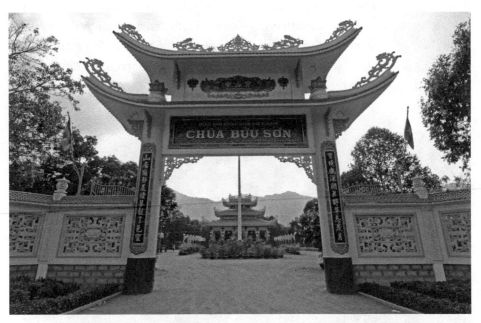

The Bửu Sơn Pagoda, sitting at the foot of the Seven Mountains

THE TWENTIETH CENTURY ONWARD

By the late 1940s, the Vietnamese Communist movement had formed into an official political party, headed by Ho Chi Minh. At this time, nationalist ideas were prevalent and modern systems of martial arts (such as the recently developed Vovinam) were utilized as tools to instill patriotic and anti-colonial ideals. Sayings were popularized that echoed these sentiments such as "Vietnamese people practice Vietnamese martial arts" and "Not a Vovinam disciple, not a patriot."[34]

During the Second Indochina War (1955-1975), practical martial arts training was widespread within the military programs and various systems (like those stemming from Binh Dinh) were adapted for military purposes by the North Vietnamese. At the same time, an array of Vietnamese and foreign combat systems were utilized by Southern forces. These include Vovinam, which already had strong foundations in the south of the country and Tae Kwon Do with up to 300,000 South Korean soldiers dispatched to South Vietnam. The Korean forces included squadrons of high-ranking martial artists and is considered to have been a major development in the spread of Tae Kwon Do both in Vietnam and in the United States.[35]

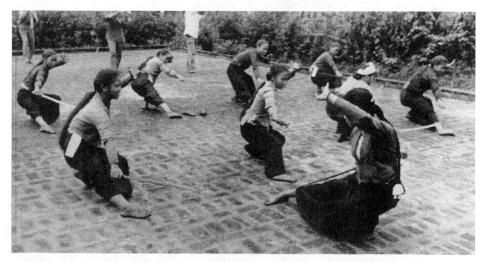

Fig. 2. A squad of Northern Vietnamese women training in martial arts (1968)

The northern *Việt Minh* army eventually took Saigon in April 1975 and officially united the country under the banner of the Socialist Republic of Vietnam. The following decade was plagued with economic and social issues, however, when the nation finally opened their borders to the outside world in the mid-1980s, there was a significant drive to develop nationalized systems of martial arts, mirroring successes in nations like Japan and Korea. This has been somewhat successful, with the development of martial arts-centered tourist areas and festivals around the country as well as the inclusion of Vovinam in the South East Asian (SEA) Games.[36]

Since the start of the new millennium, Vietnamese martial arts have continued to remain popular as sporting, self-defense, religious and cultural practices. Due in part to the strong nationalist ideals that have been instilled within Vietnamese society, historical links between the modern Viet people and ancient inhabitants of the region are often stated.[37] However, as we can see from the above, the Vietnamese martial arts are not the product of any particular group or people, but are constantly evolving cultures and traditions with a wide range of influences. While there is no definitive answer to where Vietnamese martial arts begin or end, it is safe to say that the adaptations and developments of such styles to face different landscapes, enemies and challenges throughout history certainly make them unique.

In the next chapter we will examine some of the present-day systems and styles of Vietnamese martial arts in greater detail.

CHAPTER ONE NOTES

[1] Green, Thomas A., *Martial Arts of the World: An Encyclopedia*, (Santa Barbara, CA: ABC-CLIO, 2001), 16.

[2] Taylor, K W., "Vietnamese Geopolitical Constraints," Italian Geopolitical Monthly Journal 08 (2015).

[3] Goscha, Christopher E., *The Penguin History of Modern Vietnam,* (London: Penguin Books 2017).

[4] Phạm Phong, *Lịch Sử Võ Học Việt Nam*, (Ho Chi Minh City: Nhà Xuất Bản Văn Hóa Thông Tin, 2013).

[5] Goscha, *The Penguin History*, 23.

[6] Ibid., 528.

[7] Ibid., 37.

[8] Taylor, K W., A History of the Vietnamese, (Cambridge: Cambridge University Press, 2013), 662.

[9] Ibid., 59

[10] Ngoc Huu and Lady Borton, *Martial Arts—Võ Dân Tộc*, (Hanoi, Thế Giới Publishers, 2005), 11.

[11] Goscha, *The Penguin History*, 481.

[12] Ngoc and Borton, *Martial Arts*, 31.

[13] Nguyen Manh Hung, "An Attempt to Study The Cultural History of Traditional Vietnamese Martial Arts—Section 1," The Holy Land of Vietnam Studies, September 4, 2019, http://holylandvietnamstudies.com/blog/an-attempt-to-study-the-cultural-history-of-traditional-vietnamese-martial-arts-section-1/.

[14] Ibid.

[15] Phạm, *Lịch Sử Võ*, 2013.

[16] Khai Nhan. "Báu Vật Thiêng Liêng ở Một Dòng Họ Võ." Bao Binh Dinh, September 1, 2006. http://www.baobinhdinh.com.vn/Disan-dulich/2006/9/31897/.

[17] Phạm, *Lịch Sử Võ*, 593–783.

[18] Ngoc and Borton, *Martial Arts*, 19.

[19] Cima, Ronald J and Library Of Congress, Federal Research Division. *Vietnam: A Country Study*, (Washington, D.C.: Federal Research Division, Library of Congress: 1989), https://www.loc.gov/item/88600482/, 23.

[20] Tran, Jason Hoai, "Than Quyen: An Introduction to Spirit Forms of That Son Vietnamese Martial Arts," *Journal of Asian Martial Arts* 13, no. 2 (2004): 65–78.

[21] Taylor, *A History*, 470.

[22] Dutton, George Edson, *The Tây Sơn Uprising: Society and Rebellion in Eighteenth-Century Vietnam*, (Chiang Mai, Thailand: Silkworm Books, 2008), 39.

[23] Ibid., 2.

[24] Bao Binh Dinh, "Bùi Thị Xuân," December 16, 2003, http://www.baobinhdinh.com.vn/642/2003/12/7555/.

[25] Dutton, *The Tây Sơn Uprising*, 55.

[26] Bao Binh Dinh, "Bùi Thị Xuân".

[27] Cima, *Vietnam: A Country Study*, 25.

[28] Ngoc and Borton, *Martial Arts*, 27.

[29] Green, *Martial Arts of the World*, 548.

[30] Ngoc and Borton, *Martial Arts*, 27.

[31] Goscha, *The Penguin History*, 211.

[32] Thich, Quang Huyen, *Dharma Mountain Buddhism & Martial Yoga*, (Frederick, MD: Dharma Mountain Publications, Chùa Xá Lợi 2010), 118–122.

[33] Salemink, Oscar, *The Ethnography of Vietnam's Central Highlanders: a Historical Contextualization. 1850-1990*, (Place of publication not identified: Routledge, 2019), 147.

[34] Green, *Martial Arts of the World*, 441.

[35] Gillis, Alex, *A Killing Art: The Untold History of Tae Kwon Do*, (United States: ECW Press, 2016), 82.

[36] Roe, Augustus John, "An Investigation into the Effectiveness and Relevance of Traditional Vietnamese Martial Arts," Master's Thesis, Horizons University Paris, 2019.

[37] Taylor, *A History*, 3.

CHAPTER ONE FIGURES

Figure 1.—Kyle Mathers, Tiền Giấy Mệnh Giá 200 Đồng (1966), Mặt Trước Hình Nguyễn Huệ, August 18, 2019, Wikimedia Commons. https://commons.wikimedia.org/wiki/File:200vnchA.jpg.

Figure 2.—Manh Hai, North Vietnamese ladies on martial art training, 29 April 1968, https://www.flickr.com/photos/13476480@N07/25370696725/in/photostream/.

NORTH
VIETNAMESE
STYLES
AND
SCHOOLS

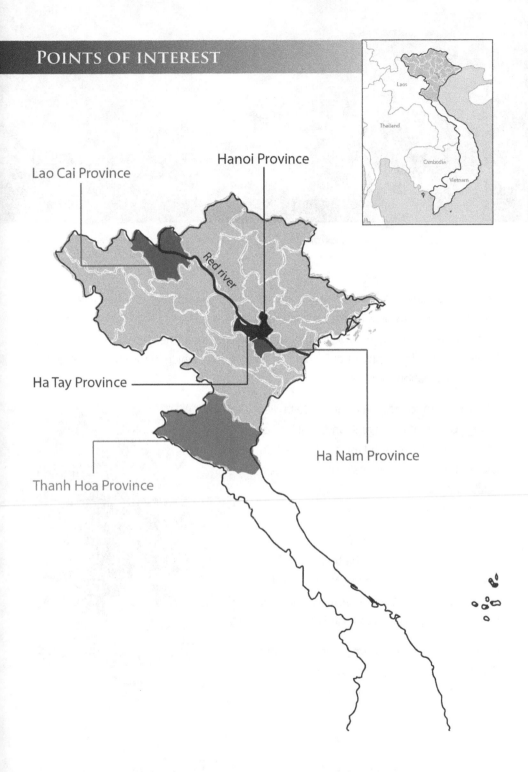

Lao Cai Province

Hanoi Province

Red river

Ha Tay Province

Ha Nam Province

Thanh Hoa Province

Laos

Thailand

Cambodia

Vietnam

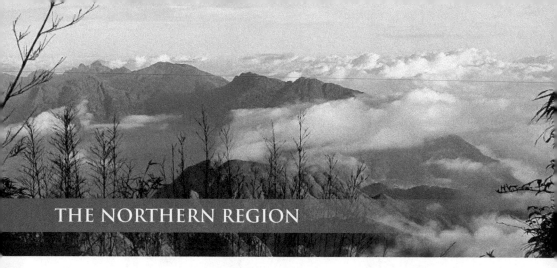

THE NORTHERN REGION

The view from Mt. Fansipan, also known as "The Roof of Indochina"

Covering an area of around fifteen thousand square kilometers is the Red River Delta, the most populous area in North Vietnam and home to the capital city of Hanoi. The Red River and its estuaries have, for thousands of years, been the lifeblood of the region, facilitating the development of farming and agriculture, which in turn has enabled the region's population to thrive.

Further north of the Red River Delta lies a range of mountainous highlands that border China to the north and Laos to the west. In Lao Cai Province lies mainland Southeast Asia's highest peak—Mount Fansipan, which stands at an elevation of 3143 meters.

These large, yet sparsely populated provinces are home to many of the nation's ethnic minority groups—the Hmong, Muong, Dai, Tay and Thai communities, among others, all inhabit this unforgiving mountainous landscape.

Formerly known as ***Thăng Long (Soaring Dragon)***, Hanoi has a population of over eight million and is the second largest city in Vietnam.

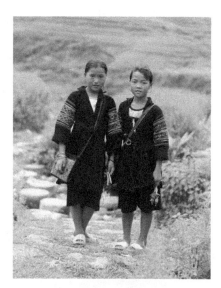

Traditionally dressed Hmong girls in Lao Cai Province

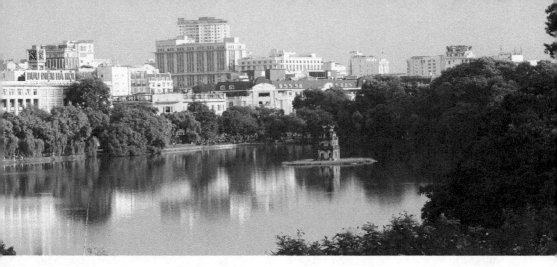

Hoan Kiem Lake features a thousand-year-old monument in the center

Although smaller than its southern counterpart, Ho Chi Minh City (formerly Saigon), Hanoi has historically been, and is still considered by many to be "the cultural and religious center, as well as the political center of the Vietnamese state."[38]

Hanoi and the surrounding provinces are also home to many important historical and geological sites, such as *Hạ Long* (literally *Descending Dragon*) Bay in Quang Ninh Province. The Bay itself is recognized by The United Nations Educational Scientific and Cultural Organization (UNESCO) as a World Heritage Site, thanks to its magnificent limestone islands, cave systems and diverse wildlife.

As we will see, there are numerous martial arts schools and styles descended from a mixture of family, military and religious lineages throughout northern Vietnam. Due to the vast but mostly uninhabitable terrain of the far north, the delta lowlands around Hanoi are home to the largest populations and as a result are known as a focal point for the development of Vietnamese martial arts.[39]

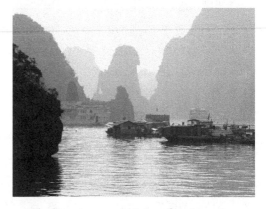

The limestone mountains of Ha Long Bay in Quang Ninh Province

Many of the northern styles of Vietnamese martial arts have been influenced by an array of sources. The Red River Delta was considered of the southernmost provinces of China for almost a thousand years, therefore Chinese influence on northern Vietnamese culture and the direction of its social-political development (including martial arts), has been extremely significant. Similarly, Khmer, Cham, Thai, Japanese and various other groups have all had a presence in the Red River Delta at certain points in history; therefore, some degree of crossover between regional cultures and martial arts would have been inevitable.

Although external influences are undeniable, many of the region's martial arts styles can be considered unique due to the ways that they have developed and adapted to suit both their environment and the physicality of their practitioners.

Beginning as long ago as the eleventh and continuing until the eighteenth century, the Royal Court was based in the ancient citadel of Thang Long and implemented martial arts examinations for military and governmental positions. These encompassed both physical and academic elements, such as the study of Confucian principles and Chinese philosophy alongside warfare and strategy. While during the second millennium, the capital city itself was a hotbed for military activity, with numerous battles and confrontations taking place within its borders

Throughout the capital city of Hanoi are hundreds of battle sites and temples devoted to honoring martial arts and famous warriors of Vietnam, some examples of which are:

- *Tháp Rùa* Temple in *Hoàn Kiếm* District. The temple is built on an island in the center of Hoan Kiem lake. It is said that the legendary warrior and Emperor, Le Loi, relinquished his sword into the waters after defeating the Ming Dynasty, claiming the throne and declaring peace.

- *Chùa Bộc* Pagoda in *Đống Đa* District. The pagoda is built on the famous site of the battle of Dong Da (1788–1789) in which Vietnamese rebels expelled invading Chinese forces from the capital.

- *Quán Thánh* Temple, in *Ba Đình* District. The temple is dedicated to the Daoist deity Tran Vu, who is known as both a protector of the city and a patron saint of warriors. As a result, many martial arts events take place here and it is seen as one of the top destinations for visitors with an interest in these aspects of Vietnam's culture.

The martial arts detailed in this chapter are some of the most popular and culturally important schools and styles in the north. They include both those widely practiced in the area today as well as those originally stemming from this region.

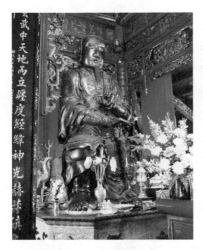
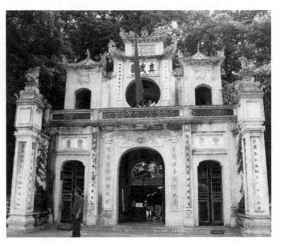

A sculptural representation of Tran Vu   *The main gate of Quan Thanh Temple in Hanoi*

NHAT NAM SCHOOL

VÕ PHÁI NHẤT NAM

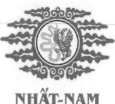

NHẤT-NAM

Fig. 3.

Võ Phái Nhất Nam translates as *One* or *First Vietnam Martial Arts*, although the meaning is not literal. The syllable *Nhất* can represent unity or modernity, while *Nam* refers to the southern kingdom, *Việt Nam.*

The provinces of Thanh Hoa and Nghe An (from which the school originate) have a long history as warring and martial states; the Tran, Le and Tay Son Dynasties all recruited numerous warriors and generals from these provinces.

As a style that takes pride in their historical roots, Nhat Nam practitioners often look to the past to draw inspiration from the courage and strength of the regions' great martial arts heroes. One example of which is Lady Trieu, often referred to as the "Vietnamese Joan of Arc,"[40] who is said to have fought off Chinese Wu Dynasty invaders from 225–248 CE.

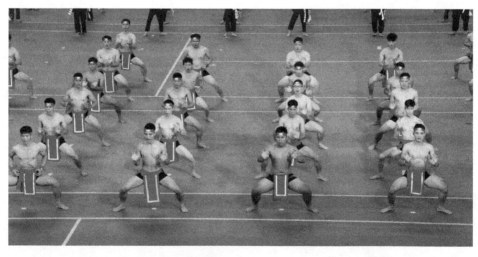

Traditionally-dressed students perform breathing drills in horse stance

HISTORY

The earliest incarnation of Nhat Nam was known as **Võ Hét** (literally *Shouting Martial Arts*). Professor Ngo Xuan Binh—the current Grandmaster of the style—states "in the ancient lands of Ai and Hoan, now known as the provinces of Thanh Hoa and Nghe An, existed a martial art used by the local people to fight wild beasts and enemies."[41]

Despite being geographically close to the Red River Delta—around two hundred kilometers south of Hanoi—Thanh Hoa and Nghe An were relatively isolated from the heavily Chinese-influenced capital to the north. What is now a several-hour drive would have historically been a massive undertaking on foot through difficult terrain.

According to Professor Ngo Xuan Binh, the style he studied was taught through successive generations of his family, often in secret due to dangerous political climates. In particular, the era following the fall of the Tay Son Dynasty demanded secretive training as it is said that during his reign, Emperor Nguyen Anh attempted to wipe out many formalized martial arts, especially among those that had collaborated with the Tay Son Rebellion.[42]

Binh began training in the style at a young age under family members and local masters from both Thanh Hoa and Nghe An. Eventually, he used his connections to unite several traditional branches of Vo Het and on October 23, 1983, the first Nhat Nam martial arts school officially opened in Hanoi.

Currently, the Nhat Nam School operates throughout Vietnam, but remains most popular in Hanoi, Thanh Hoa and Nghe An Provinces. There are also thousands of international Nhat Nam practitioners worldwide, with schools operating in dozens of cities throughout Eastern Europe, the United Kingdom, France and others.

Besides martial arts, Professor Ngo Xuan Binh is also a poet, author, traditional medicine expert and lecturer who has published multiple books on a variety of subjects. Binh teaches regular seminars in Vietnam and Europe with students traveling from all over the world to attend.

CHARACTERISTICS

Due to its origins in agricultural communities, many natural aspects are incorporated into the practice of Nhat Nam martial arts. As Binh states "this martial art is based on nature. Ancient people studied the attributes of both flora and fauna, and their natural surroundings."[43]

Common techniques of the Nhat Nam style include tiger-claw hand strikes, rooster-kicks (quick attacks that thrust with the heel, reminiscent of the animal), and grappling based upon the coiling and twisting motions of a snake. These are reflected in the Nhat Nam emblem with a snake and rooster fighting in the heart of the image. The image is also said to represent the hard and soft or Yin and Yang elements of Daoist traditions, which are key principles of the fighting style.[44]

Master Tran Ha Manh describes the typical progression of learning within the style as: flexibility and stance training, pair blocking and evasion drills, forms, practical applications of the forms and finally sparring (live fighting practice). After mastering basic forms, students are also trained in the use of traditional weapons such as staffs and swords. Master Tran also notes that as Vietnamese practitioners are typically small in stature, weight and height advantages are regarded as less important than technical skills— non-linear movements and quick evasions are emphasized to ensure practitioners have the best chances of success during conflict.[45]

Master Tran also notes that as Vietnamese practitioners are typically small in stature; weight and height advantages are regarded as less important than technical skills— non-linear movements and quick evasions are emphasized to ensure practitioners have the best chances of success during conflict.

In "Nhat Nam Martial Arts: Volume One," Professor Ngo Xuan Binh explains the key principles of the style as written below:

- "To seek for quality, not quantity.

- To understand a lot, to act precisely.

- To seek for essence, not for form; when you seize the form, do not forget that the essence hides behind the surface.

- Will and courage are more important than consideration.

- Action comes from the consciousness.

- First, you must strengthen your will and courage, later seek for mastery.

- First, understand, and then act.

- If you want to defend yourself, you have to understand how to attack.

- If you want to attack, you have to know how to defend.

- Knowing how to defend and attack are the preconditions of winning."[46]

Standard uniforms of the Nhat Nam school are sleeveless red and black tops and trousers. For performances and demonstrations, students occasionally wear the traditional attire of a red loincloth and bandanna. The uniforms vary depending on rank and school, but generally do not feature belt systems like many formalized schools of martial arts; however, masters of the style often wear white, which is said to symbolize purity and light.[47]

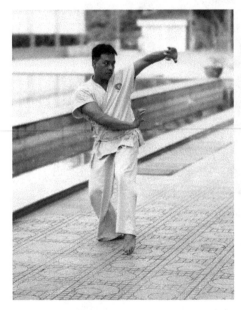 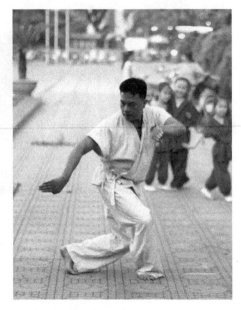

Master Tran Ha Manh performs tiger claw and snake techniques

Benefits of Nhat nam training

- Breath control: Nhat Nam utilizes a specific technique of deep, guttural breathing that is combined with shouts and vocalizations. This is said to assist with lending explosive energy to the strikes through the use of abdominal muscles, core strength and the coordination of breathing and motion.

- Applications for self-defense: Nhat Nam is a style focused on practicality and the types of techniques taught emphasize this. Examples include dual strikes (hitting with both hands, elbows, arms and legs simultaneously to ensure maximum damage) and groundwork—emphasis placed upon rolling, tripping and defense from the floor against standing opponents.[48]

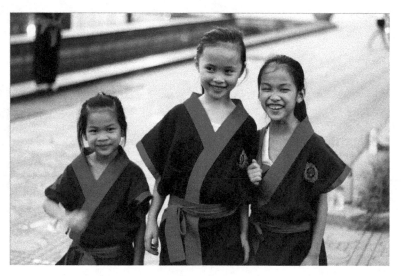

Young students in standard Nhat Nam uniforms

VIETNAMESE TRADITIONAL WRESTLING
ĐẤU VẬT

In many cultures throughout the globe, local styles of wrestling have developed as forms of sport, entertainment and combat training.[49] Vietnamese traditional wrestling, or *Đấu Vật*, has followed a similar path. It is most commonly practiced in festivals for the Lunar New Year, or Tet, within famous "wrestling villages" such as Lieu Doi Village, Ha Nam Province and Lai An Village, Phu Vang District, in Hue.

Besides its use within festivals, Dau Vat remains trained as a modern competitive sport (similar to freestyle wrestling), while aspects of the style have also been incorporated into many other systems of Vietnamese martial arts.

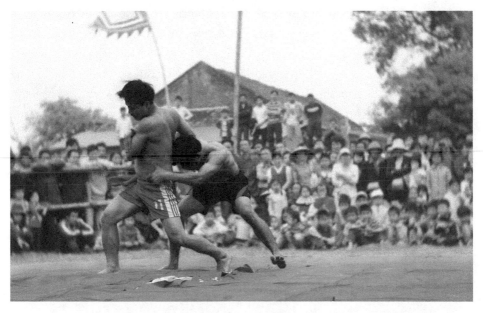

Wrestlers in a traditional bout in Lieu Doi Village

HISTORY

According to the village elders of Lieu Doi, a renowned wrestling village in Ha Nam Province (about sixty kilometers southwest of Hanoi), the origins of their style first developed over a thousand years ago.[50]

It is said that the founder, known only as Doan, was going about his work as a farmhand just outside the village boundaries when a flash flood ravaged the area causing panic among locals. Doan immediately ran from the field to give aid and as he got close to the village center, he came across a glowing sword resting on a red cloth in the surrounding rice paddy. Doan instantly realized that he had received a sacred gift and tied the sword around his waist with the red cloth.

In the years following his find, war came to the nation and the strongest fighters of each village were called upon to defend the country from invaders. Doan saw his opportunity; he enlisted in the military and quickly developed a reputation as a fierce warrior. Before battles he would cover himself with the sacred earth from the village in which his weapon was discovered. According to the story, Doan's divine gifts brought him supernatural strength and skills while the earth covering his skin protected him from spears and swords. Through the years, Doan taught many local citizens the skills he developed in combat and trained them in methods for defeating assailants armed with a sword or spear while unarmed themselves. This martial prowess of the local inhabitants is said to have ensured the prosperity of the region and earned them a reputation as warriors.

Eventually, after many long years in the military and protecting his homelands, Doan was killed in battle. He left behind his wife Bui, who as the legend goes, died of overwhelming grief after visiting Doan's final resting place. The pair were then immortalized in two shrines placed a few hundred meters apart from each other just outside Lieu Doi Village.

In modern times, Doan and Bui are seen as god-like figures protecting the citizens of this sacred region, they are affectionately referred to as *Thánh Ông* and *Tiên Bà* (literally *God* and *Goddess*) and have been celebrated in Dau Vat contests ever since.

It is claimed that local archives, dating back hundreds of years, record Doan as a legitimate historical figure. However, as with many legends, facts tend to blend with fiction, as stories are naturally embellished.

Every two years, Lieu Doi Village holds a wrestling festival on the fifth day of the Lunar New Year. The locals view this tradition not just as a fighting contest or a show of athleticism, but as an integral part of their heritage. Anyone able-bodied is encouraged to wrestle as doing so brings prosperity for the coming year and honor to one's family and ancestors.[51]

The festival begins with a parade of thousands trailing out from the centuries old *Sới Vật* (or *Wrestling Arena*) toward the long, single dirt road leading into the village. As they reach the shrine of the legendary *Thánh Ông*, village elders perform a ritual of burning incense and delivering gifts, then pray for the blessings of the local deities to hold the festival and provide luck for the coming year. The festival officially begins with a reenactment of Doan, played by one of the most highly-respected village elders, finding the sacred sword and cloth, which is followed by a flag dance to the beat of a ritual drum.

Citizens from the surrounding four hamlets take their places around the wrestling ring—a ripped and worn canvas tarpaulin placed on beds of straw and rice husks. The first few bouts are symbolic, one of which, known as *Trai Rốt* (or *Final Boy*), requires the sons of villagers born on the most auspicious dates of the previous year to wrestle in an exhibition match. This is obviously impractical, due to the sons being at most one year old; therefore, fathers and even grandfathers fight on their behalf.

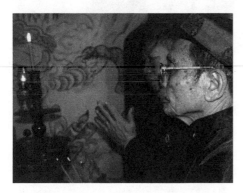

Lieu Doi Village elders
praying to Thanh Ong and Tien Ba

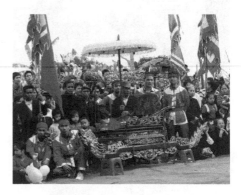

Palanquin bearers
waiting for the contest to begin

In the following contests, competitors are eliminated one by one until a single fighter remains. The final round then consists of five back-to-back fights; the winner sits in the center of the ring wearing a symbolic red scarf and takes on any five challengers who step forward.

If the champion remains victorious in all successive bouts, it is said that he brings great prosperity to the village and is presented with "Doan's" red cloth, ceremonial sword and a sprig of bamboo which symbolizes the new life of spring.

The traditions of Dau Vat have been passed on through family lineages for generations. It is seen as a birthright for children from the region to learn to wrestle and they often do so from a very young age. However, the village-elders of Lieu Doi identify the increasing migration of young practitioners from their villages to the big cities in search of opportunity, as a threat to the ongoing practice of Dau Vat. Fortunately, there are groups of dedicated martial artists in Lieu Doi and other famous wrestling villages who strive to ensure their style continues.

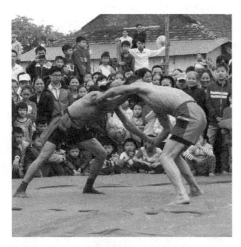

A father and grandfather wrestling in the symbolic Trai Rot rounds

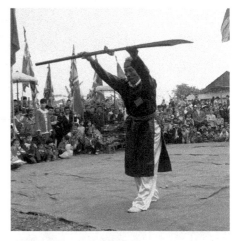

*The opening ceremony –
A village elder pays tribute to Thanh Ong*

CHARACTERISTICS

Through the author's own experiences participating in Lieu Doi's traditional wrestling festival, alongside interviews with a number of wrestlers within the village, it can be pertained that the following characteristics are uniform throughout the practice of Dau Vat:

- Fights begin with a short ceremony. The opponents come to the center of the mat and perform venerations to their ancestors—this takes the form of prayers and a dance-like routine that invokes both spiritual power while also serving as a warm up, similar to the *Wai Kru* in Muay Thai.[52] Fighters then shake hands and when instructed by the referee and begin.

- The style of fighting is rapid, involving short rounds that run for up to two minutes. This helps to ensure that the contests are undertaken with maximum speed and force.

- Competitors must uproot their opponents through throws, trips, sweeps and takedowns.

- To win, wrestlers must make both of their opponent's shoulders touch the ground simultaneously or take both of their feet from the mat. Losing balance or falling like this is considered to leave a fighter exposed to further attacks in a battle situation.

- Striking is disallowed. However, there are non-competitive forms still practiced that permit strikes.

- Various techniques maintain historical relevance. Certain positions are avoided due to vulnerability against opponents bearing swords and there are several high-level grabs and throws said to have been adapted from taking charging attackers off horseback.

- Wrestling festivals typically run for three days and each competitor has at least six matches.

- Winners are often awarded small monetary prizes; however, the *real* prize is thought to be the honor and prosperity the competitors earn for their families in the coming year.

Although there is no official uniform for Dau Vat, fighters often wrestle shirtless wearing red or blue shorts. Historically, wrestlers were required to wear only a loincloth; however, this tradition has been updated for practicality and modern aesthetic value.

Benefits of Dau Vat training

- Explosive power: Due to short rounds, Dau Vat matches are fast paced and favor explosive throwing techniques rather than extended grapples. Training in this manner may offer similar benefits for practitioners of other grappling styles.

- Footwork and speed: There are very few weight classes in Dau Vat contests, therefore emphasis is placed on quick-movement and footwork which allows lighter competitors to overcome those with more mass and muscular strength.

- Application: Due to the widespread, global nature of wrestling, techniques taught in Dau Vat may be easily applied to other forms of grappling and vice-versa.

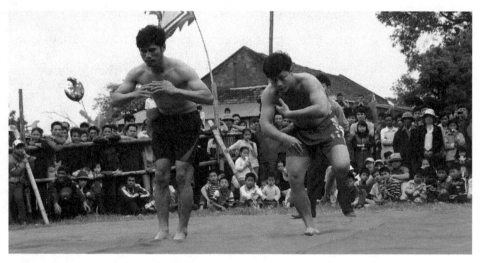

Two wrestlers perform pre-fight venerations during the New Year festival in Lieu Doi Village

NAM HONG SON SCHOOL

VÕ PHÁI NAM HỒNG SƠN

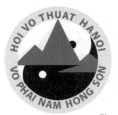

Fig. 4.

Võ Phái Nam Hồng Sơn is one of the largest martial arts styles practiced in the north of Vietnam, with thousands of students across dozens of schools. *Võ Phái* means *style*, *Nam* represents *Vietnam*, *Hồng* is taken from *Hồng Gia Quyền* (*Hung Gar Kuen*), which influenced the system and *Sơn*, meaning *Mountain*, represents the spirit of the martial arts, which is solid yet majestic.[53]

Due to the development of Nam Hong Son in the early twentieth century from a combination of Chinese and Viet influences, in the author's opinion, the style can be considered as a Sino-Vietnamese martial art.

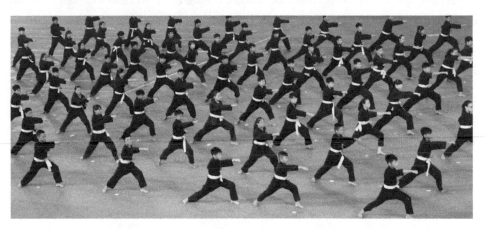

Students perform techniques at a festival of traditional martial arts in Hanoi

History

The school's founder. Nguyen Van To, was born in 1895 in Bach Dang village, Ha Tay Province. He and his family are said to have lived peacefully until one day when their village was attacked by a band of criminals.

As a result of losing nearly everything they owned, Nguyen Van To decided to learn martial arts to protect his family and his fellow villagers. Eventually, he moved to Hanoi to live with his brother and found work for a French company making tires. Nguyen Van To then began to study a style of Shaolin Hung Gar Kuen—at the time this was strictly prohibited by the ruling French government and had to be practiced in total secrecy. After several years of training he decided to expand his knowledge by studying the traditional martial arts styles of Vietnam. Through luck and dedication, he managed to track down three famous master-brothers known as Cu Ba Cat, Cu Cu Ton and Cu Han Bai—*Cu* meaning great-grandfather or in this case, patriarch master.

After getting to know the brothers, working alongside them and earning their trust Van To was eventually accepted as a "family member," which meant he was permitted to study their style (at the time martial arts were usually kept within family lineages). After the French occupation ended and Vietnam began to further open up as a nation, Master Nguyen Van To, supported by his "brothers," decided to open a school. The founders together decided upon the name Nam Hong Son.

The first formal school was founded in 1920 in Hai Ba Trung District, downtown Hanoi. After operating for many years, it was destroyed by a bomb blast in 1948—an all too common sign of the turbulent era. During the period of war with the French, Grandmaster Nguyen Van To trained many high-ranking military officers and generals in martial arts. This helped spread the name and reputation of the system and its students.[54]

Grandmaster Nguyen Van To passed away in 1984, leaving over three hundred masters across Vietnam.[55] Nguyen Van Ty, the Grandmaster's son, is the current head of the organization, which is based in Hanoi, while a number of both Vietnamese and foreign masters operate schools throughout Europe and the United States.

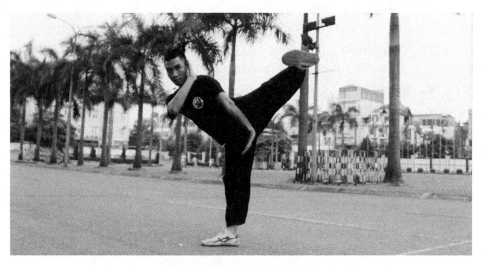

A mid-range kick and groin block

CHARACTERISTICS

The Nam Hong Son style was developed as a "smooth and flexible combination of both Vietnamese and Chinese martial arts traditions." [56]

Instructor Le Trung Linh summarizes the features of the style to be quick transitions between high-level hand strikes and low-level kicks (suitable for small-statured practitioners) and the use of non-linear angles and circular evasions. While the major differences between Nam Hong Son and Hung Gar Kuen include the frequent use of jumping and high kicks, fast successions of open-handed strikes and the inclusion of several Binh Dinh style forms within practice. This variety of techniques is considered to provide students of Nam Hong Son with more flexibility than their Hung Gar Kuen counterparts. [57]

Typical classes consist of strength and flexibility exercises, striking and self-defense drills, competitive fighting practice and form training (set sequences of attacking and defensive movements that include empty-handed techniques, animal styles and weapons). Three of the core forms trained in the Nam Hong Son system are: *Khai Tâm Quyền* (*Opening-The-Mind Form*), *Long Hổ Quyền* (*Dragon-Tiger Form*) and *Tứ Lộ Đoản Quyền* (*The Short Four-Way Form*).

Demonstrations of Nam Hong Son often feature displays of "hard-body conditioning" (literally training parts of the body to receive extreme forces or blows with minimal damage, reminiscent of their Shaolin counterparts). These include bending steel bars with the limbs or head, motorbikes being driven over practitioners' chests, and bricks being smashed using various body parts.[58]

Nguyen Van Ty describes the central tenants of the Nam Hong Son philosophy as the following:

- "You must be respectful to teachers and classmates; they are to be treated as brothers.

- Martial arts must never be taught to those who will use them for bad purposes.

- One should be humble and learn with humility and devotion.

- Martial arts should only be used for defense and never with bad intent.

- Students must use their skills to unite against evil and be ready to defend their country and principles."[59]

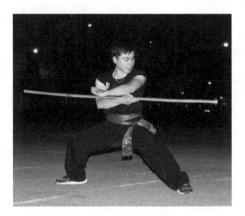 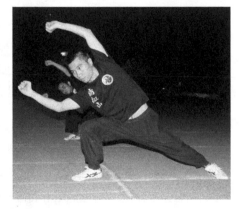

Master Le Trung Linh and a student demonstrating staff and open-hand techniques

The ranking system of the Nam Hong Son School differs from many other traditional Vietnamese martial arts styles. Instead of growing from darker to lighter shades as the practitioner progresses, belts run: white, black, blue, green, yellow and red. Red belt is the highest rank available and ranges from levels one to eight, while level nine is reserved for Grandmasters. Students typically wear black pants and long-sleeved shirts adorned with the school logo.

Benefits of Nam Hong Son Training

- Well-rounded skills: The Nam Hong Son style emphasizes variety; students are encouraged to develop striking, weapons, self-defense skills, fitness and traditional aspects, such as form.

- Combat sport training: The organization includes a syllabus of full-contact combat sport fighting (similar in rules to Chinese Sanda) and regularly holds competitions across the country.

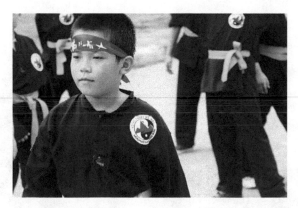

Young students prepare to display their martial arts skills

VOVINAM

VIET VO DAO/VIÊT VÕ ĐẠO

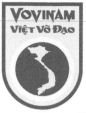

Fig. 5.

The largest and most easily recognizable style of Vietnamese martial arts is Vovinam or **Việt Võ Đạo**, with an estimated one-and-a-half million practitioners across five continents.[60] Vovinam comes from the words **Võ** (literally **fighting**) and **Nam** (meaning **Vietnam**) pushed together. Whereas a more recent adaptation of the name, **Việt Võ Đạo**, translates as **The Way of Vietnamese Martial Arts**.

Vovinam is one of Vietnam's national sports and is rapidly becoming recognized worldwide as a highly-respected style of East Asian martial arts. This is displayed through its official inclusion as one of thirty-six sports within the Southeast Asian (SEA) Games.

Vovinam was officially formed in Hanoi, although the world headquarters are now based in Ho Chi Minh City. The style maintains a wide following throughout the entire length of the country.

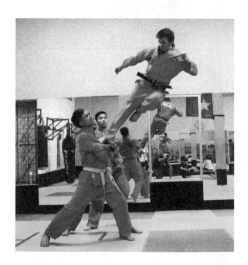 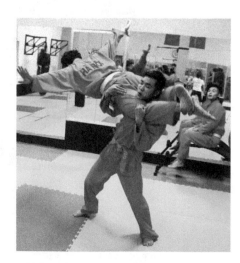

Master Bui Tuan Dat and his students
demonstrate some of the famous aerial techniques of Vovinam

History

Vovinam was officially founded in 1938 by the late Grandmaster Nguyen Loc, a resident of Hanoi. As a child Nguyen Loc was encouraged to study various Vietnamese and foreign martial arts by his parents as a way wanted to make sure he was able to stay healthy and defend himself.

After some time, Nguyen Loc began to combine the techniques he had learned from traditional Vietnamese styles along with Chinese and Japanese systems, creating an efficient and practical martial art which he viewed as being "compatible with the modern culture and state of mind of people of his generation."[61]

In 1940, Loc and a small number of students were invited to demonstrate Vovinam at the Hanoi Opera House. Their performance was reported to be hugely successful and attracted many supporters).[62] As a result, Loc was asked to begin teaching at *Hanoi Ecole Normale* (Hanoi University of Education). During this period, Vovinam gained a strong nationalist following and built a solid foundation for its future use as a device to assist in aggregating the Vietnamese people.[63]

Following these developments, Vovinam was soon identified as being a factor in developing anti-French sentiment and prohibited by the government. In response, the system was taught in secret for a number of years, then following the French expulsion from Vietnam, Grandmaster Nguyen Loc moved to Saigon and in 1955, finally opened Vovinam's first official training center.

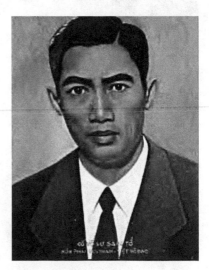

Fig. 6. Patriarch Master—Nguyen Loc

Although it was developed with the intent of being a self-defense tool, a key tenet of early Vovinam was patriotism as it provided "a focus for national identity for the Vietnamese people."[64]

Grandmaster Nguyen Loc had seen these ideals displayed in other martial arts; Japan had Judo, Korea had Taekwondo and Vietnam could now find a similar sense of pride with Vovinam.

Despite periods of conflict, Vovinam developed steadily both in terms of practitioners and global recognition during the latter half of the twentieth century. After Nguyen Loc's death in 1960, the development of Vovinam was continued by his successor, the late Grandmaster Le Sang, then by Grandmaster Nguyen Van Chieu until his death in 2020. Currently there are Vovinam schools in more than fifty countries across Asia, Europe, North and South America, Australia and Africa.

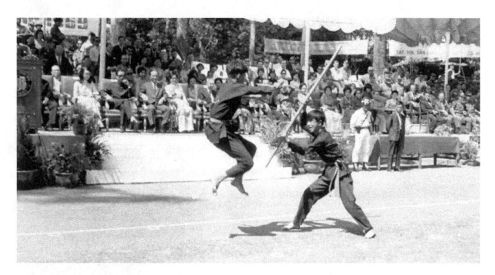

Fig. 7. A demonstration of Viet Vo Dao in Dao Tan Park, Ho Chi Minh City during the 1970s

CHARACTERISTICS

Vovinam is a diverse and dynamic martial art that fuses traditional and modern styles into a practical package. As Nguyen Hung, vice-president of the French Federation of Vovinam-Viet Vo Dao, states "with its wide variety of techniques, Vovinam is the complete martial art."[65]

Hanoi-based Master of Vovinam, Bui Tuan Dat, describes the key attributes of the style as the following:

- Dynamic high and low attacks. For example, its system of twenty-one low kicks and "flying scissor" takedowns—in which practitioners leap up and wrap their legs around an opponent's neck using momentum to send them flying. According to Tran "tradition holds that these maneuvers were developed in the thirteenth century as a means to allow Vietnamese foot soldiers to attack Mongol cavalrymen."[66]

- Fast and aggressive knees and elbows, typical of other Southeast Asian martial arts such as Muay Thai and Cambodian *Bokator*.

- Grappling and throws developed from systems such as Judo and Vietnamese Traditional Wrestling.

- Weapons training. Long and short staffs, swords and halberds are all practiced and students sometimes train with knives and small blades reminiscent of Malay, Indonesian or Filipino styles of martial arts.

- Competitive fighting. This system uses kickboxing-style rules, but also awards points for throws and takedowns.[67]

In terms of philosophy, the "Hard-Soft" (Yin/Yang) principle of Vovinam is considered to be key.[68] This is displayed in the Vovinam logo which is based upon the symbol with a map of Vietnam in the center and the two largest cities, Hanoi and Ho Chi Minh City over the poles. It is also demonstrated in the martial elements of the system, which emphasizes both relaxed and supple (soft) techniques alongside linear strikes and (hard) techniques similar to those found in Karate.

Vovinam has a strong code of ethics and etiquette that, to the observer, appears reminiscent of Japanese and Korean martial arts. However, in contrast to some traditional martial arts, Vovinam is a progressive system that actively encourages students to "research and innovate new martial arts' techniques to improve Vovinam-Viet Vo Dao's technical resources."[69]

In summary, Vovinam is a well-rounded and complete system. It is one of the few Vietnamese martial arts that covers everything from weapons and stand-up fighting to grappling and groundwork. This holistic approach to combat may have been a significant reason for Vovinam's successes in the early years of its inception.

Vovinam uniforms are based upon the Japanese *Gi* (the training outfit often used in Karate and Judo schools) but are light blue in color as opposed to the traditional white. The belt ranking system works through a progression of colors: beginners wear light blue; students wear a darker blue; instructors from first to fourth *Đẳng* (equivalent to the Japanese *Dan* system in which several levels of black belt are awarded) wear yellow; fourth to tenth *Đẳng* Masters wear red with white stripes indicating specific ranks and the Grandmaster wears white.

The color schemes of Vovinam belts are said to represent the skill sets that develop: blue represents the ocean and the depth of martial arts study; yellow is said to represent the earth in which roots grow, indicating the depth of the student's knowledge; red represents fire or blood indicating the martial arts skill of the practitioner; and white as the top rank represents infinity.

Benefits of Vovinam training

- Fitness: Due to a focus on competition and the incorporation of modern training methodologies, Vovinam provides excellent all-round exercise with a mix of cardiovascular conditioning, flexibility, endurance and strength training.

- Practicality: The combative roots of the style emphasize a direct teaching methodology. As Tran states, in contrast to many traditional Chinese combatives "forms are readily understandable by any student and can be used immediately."[70]

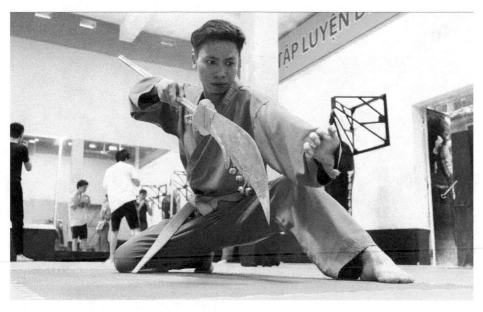

An instructor demonstrates a combined Halberd and Tiger-Claw technique

THANH PHONG SCHOOL

VÕ ĐƯỜNG THANH PHONG

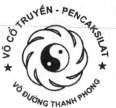

Fig. 8.

The Thang Phong School teaches a modern hybrid-system of traditional Vietnamese arts, but also incorporates aspects of Pencak Silat, Hung Gar Kuen, Wing Chun and others. In recent years, the school has amassed a large following in and around the capital city thanks to the straightforward teaching style and charisma of founder Master Hoang Thanh Phong.

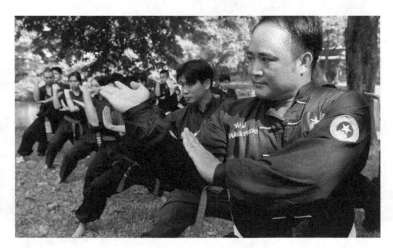

Fig. 9. Master Thanh Phong leading form practice in a suburb of Hanoi

HISTORY

According to Master Hoang, he began learning traditional Vietnamese martial arts in the 1960s and in his youth also studied various Chinese and Southeast Asian martial arts under a number of renowned foreign and Vietnamese masters. He was eventually awarded one of the highest ranks in *Võ Cổ Truyền* (the umbrella term for Binh Dinh region martial arts).

In 1985, aged twenty-one, Master Hoang opened his first school on Quang Trung Street in Hanoi. He began teaching an amalgamated system of Vietnamese and foreign martial arts, taking what he deemed to be the most valuable aspects of each style and soon earned himself a solid reputation within the martial arts community.

In 1991, Master Hoang was invited to train the national Pencak Silat team and over the next three years Vietnamese Pencak Silat practitioners went on to win seven medals at the Southeast Asian Games as well as three world championships. In 2008, the Thang Phong School was officially recognized by the UNESCO heritage committee for contributing to the conservation of the oriental martial arts.[71]

Alongside martial arts, the Thanh Phong School also trains students for festival performances of Lion Dance and various other martial-arts centered activities. For example, one student, ten-year-old Hoang Gia Khoa broke the national record by pulling a three-ton car with his neck for a distance of 143 meters.[72]

There are currently over fifty schools in the capital city and surrounding provinces with students numbering in the thousands.[73] Master Thang Phong teaches both publicly and works with branches of the military and police force delivering seminars on self-defense and combat techniques.

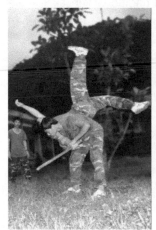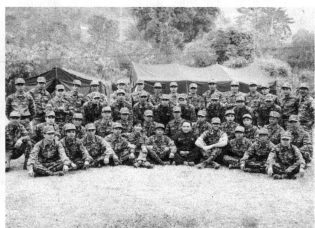

Fig. 10-11. Master Thang Phong training with the Vietnamese military

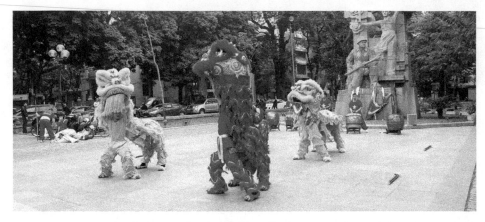

Fig. 12. Thanh Phong School students performing a Lion Dance in Hanoi

Although the Thanh Phong School syllabus has been developed primarily from traditional Vietnamese martial arts, various other Asian systems have all made significant contributions.

Master Hoang considers the key strength of his school to be their empty-handed techniques. However, his syllabus also includes a range of traditional weapons and hard-body conditioning similar to Shaolin Kung Fu (such as practitioners breaking bricks with their fists). Meanwhile, some self-defense principles of traditional Pencak Silat are incorporated, such as an emphasis on the training of bladed weapons and practice in defending against attackers bearing knives.[74]

The Thanh Phong School teaches classes in military-like formations, with students moving through forms and techniques in unison while arranged in lines, similar to other foreign arts such as Karate and Taekwondo. Master Hoang says "this method helps to instill the discipline required in younger students and make for a quick and effective way of learning."[75]

Although developed from a combination of Vietnamese and foreign arts, one unique aspect of the Thanh Phong School is its focus on the advancement of Vietnam and Vietnamese principles. According to Master Hoang:

"The school aims to develop three key areas: the first is the spirit of the Vietnamese people; the second is the strength and patriotism of its practitioners; and the third is the health of the nation so that they can further their own development."[76]

The six guiding principles of the Thanh Phong martial arts school state that students must:

- "Respect their seniors and peers
- Be peaceful and modest
- Maintain discipline and unity
- Abide by the law and its teachings
- Never belittle others or show arrogance
- Not do dishonorable deeds ."[77]

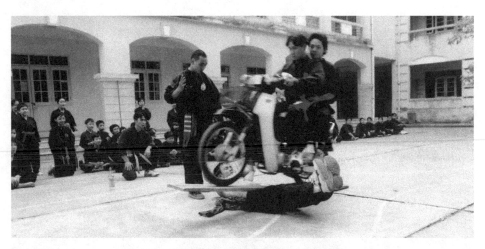

Fig. 13. A student demonstrates "hard-body" conditioning by having a motocycle driven over his chest

Students typically wear black button-up shirts and long pants with a blue, yellow, red or white sash indicating their status as a beginner, student, teacher or master. However, since the school highlights patriotism as one of their key principles, performance clothes are often bright red and adorned with the yellow star of the Vietnamese flag.

Benefits of Thanh Phong School training

- Discipline and Focus: Mental training is one of the major selling points of the style. This has likely worked toward cementing the Thanh Phong School's reputation as one of the leading clubs for children and teens to study martial arts in north Vietnam.

- Adaptability: The combination of traditional and modern elements means the school provides a solid all-round program that encompasses self-defense, fitness, mental training and philosophy.

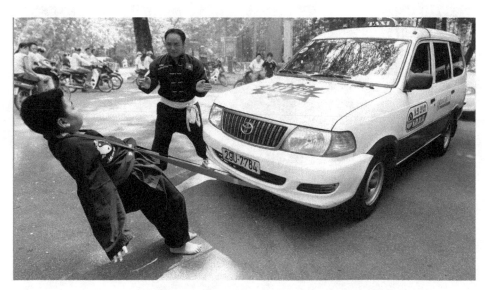

Fig. 14. Master and student during the record breaking attempt

THE BAC VIET VO SCHOOL

Võ Đường Bắc Việt Võ

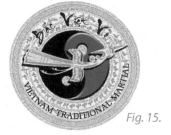

Fig. 15.

The name ***Bắc Việt Võ*** literally means ***Northern Vietnam Martial Arts*** and is one of particular interest due to the background of their style, coming from Hmong practices rather than those of the Viet people.

Whilst the Hmong, make up less than two percent of the overall population, they reside in much greater proportions in the northern highlands and some highland areas of Nghe An Province. In recent years, the Bac Viet Vo School, based in Lao Cai Province, has amassed a solid following of both Hmong and Viet practitioners. This may be due to the flexible yet practical nature of the style, the allure of a system which has historically never been shared with outsiders or a combination of the two.

HISTORY

Throughout history, many of Vietnam's minority groups have faced tremendous hardships, living in deadly landscapes, filled with wild animals and simultaneously facing regular conflict and persecution from various ruling factions. As a result, the development of self-defense techniques in the rugged north can be considered to have born out of necessity.[78]

Although it is thought that the Hmong (a sub-group of the Miao people) have inhabited the Yellow River region of China for thousands of years, unlike most of the other groups in the region, they did not venture southwards until the eighteenth century when "as many as 10,000 are recorded arriving in Vietnam."[79]

While it is only possible to speculate as to the martial history of the Hmong people in the Yellow River region of China, it is known that a variety of weapons such as the machete and crossbow were widely utilized by the historical inhabitants and it is likely that there would have been cultural crossover with their ethnic Chinese cohabitants. Furthermore, during the migration into Northern Vietnam during a turbulent era, it is entirely possible that the Hmong groups encountered Vietnamese martial arts traditions along the way.

The Hmong martial arts were relatively unknown to the majority of Vietnamese people until recent years, however in the past decade, Master Tran Ngoc Linh from Lao Cai Province has established schools of his family clan's style in Hanoi, Lao Cai and several other locations throughout the north of the country.

Master Tran claims that many clans like his own, maintain their own relatively distinct fighting systems which have previously been taught only behind closed doors.[80]

CHARACTERISTICS

To the observer, the Hmong styles appear aesthetically different from many of the common Viet systems. For example, rather than "stepping through" between stances, they often utilize hops or jumps, this type of movement may be better suited to the features of a rocky and mountainous terrain. Furthermore, within the Bac Viet Vo style of martial arts, the majority of weapons practiced are farming or hunting tools (rather than battle-weapons), such as the machete, daggers, and the use of crossbow and quiver as both projectile and striking tools.[81]

Other key features are the incorporation of diagonal and horizontal open-handed attacks, which can be used interchangeably as striking blows, parrying/blocking techniques or in close range to lock opponents' joints. It is said that this method of combined attack and defense is favored due to its effective and uncomplicated applications.[82]

Students of the Bac Viet Vo School typically wear traditional ethnic outfits. For everyday practices they may be simple black or dark blue cotton shirts and pants, while for performances or demonstrations more decorative attire with woven multicolored or gold-thread patterns may be worn.

Benefits of Bac Viet Vo Training

- Balance and stability: Due to the practices of the style that often take place on uneven and rocky terrain, these aspects are heavily emphasized within training.

- Culture: The ethnic background of the art offers insight into a different people from many of the Viet martial arts. As a result, aspects of Hmong culture such as language, history or religious/spiritual practices are all featured within the practices of the Bac Viet Vo style.

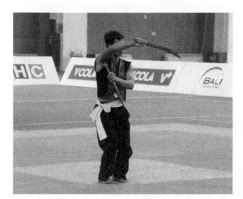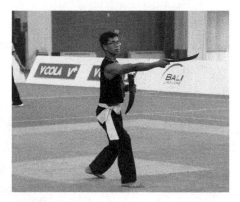

Instructor Dang Lai from the Bac Viet Vo School demonstrates a machete form

CHAPTER TWO NOTES

[38] Logan, William Stewart, *Hanoi: Biography of a City*, (Sydney: University of New South Wales Press, 2000), 25.

[39] Ngoc Huu and Lady Borton, *Martial Arts—Võ Dân Tộc*, (Hanoi, Thế Giới Publishers, 2005), 29.

[40] Keri Lynn Engel, "Trieu Thi Trinh, the Vietnamese Joan of Arc," Amazing Women In History, March 1, 2012, https://amazingwomeninhistory.com/trieu-thi-trinh-the-vietnamese-joan-of-arc/.

[41] Hoang Hieu Trung, "Martial Arts Maketh the Man," vietnamnews.vn, Viet Nam News, January 22, 2012, https://vietnamnews.vn/Sunday/Features/220019/martial-arts-maketh-the-man.html.

[42] Ibid., para. 12.

[43] Ibid., para. 9.

[44] Nhat Nam U.K., "Nhat Nam School Philosophy," 2018, http://nhat-nam.co.uk/philosophy/.

[45] Tran Ha Manh, Master of Nhat Nam Style, in discussion with the author, Viet-Xo Friendship Palace, 91 Tran Hung Dao, Hai Ba Trung District, Hanoi, June 2015.

[46] Ngo, Binh Xuan, *Nhất Nam Căn Bản 1*, (Hanoi: Thế Giới Publishers, 2010).

[47] Tran, in discussion with the author, 2015.

[48] Ngo, *Nhất Nam Căn Bản*, 364-385.

[49] lanchard, Kendall, *The Anthropology of Sport: an Introduction*, (Westport, CT: Bergin & Garvey, 1995), 101.

[50] Lieu Doi Village Elders Committee, In discussion with the author, Lieu Doi Village, Liem Tuc Commune, Thanh Liem District, Ha Nam Province. February 2014.

[51] Ngoc and Borton, *Martial Arts*, 51.

[52] Green, Thomas A., *Martial Arts of the World: An Encyclopedia*, (Santa Barbara, CA: ABC-CLIO, 2001), 352.

53 Truong Van Bao, "Võ Sư Nguyễn Nguyên Tộ Và Môn Phái Nam Hồng Sơn," Liên Đoàn Võ Thuật Cổ Truyền Việt Nam, August 12, 2015, http://vocotruyenvietnam.vn/van-hoa-vo-thuat/ton-vinh/vo-su-nguyen-nguyen-to-va-mon-phai-nam-hong-son.aspx.

54 Nguyen Van Ty, "Lịch Sử Môn Phái Nam Hồng Sơn," www.namhongson.vn, October 1, 2010, http://namhongson.vn/02/01/Lich-su-mon-phai-Nam-Hong-Son.htm.

55 Truong, "Võ Sư Nguyễn Nguyên Tộ," 2015.

56 Ngoc and Borton, *Martial Arts*, 27.

57 Le Trung Linh, Nam Hong Son Instructor, in discussion with the author, Quan Ngua Stadium, Ba Dinh District, Hanoi, May 2016.

58 Van Bich, "Xuan Duc Martial Arts Club," Vietnam Pictorial, April 15, 2014, https://vietnam.vnanet.vn/english /xuan-duc-martial-arts-club/59518.html.

59 Nguyen, "Lịch Sử Môn Phái," 2010, para. 18.

60 Matthew Knight and Natasha Maguder, "Nguyen Van Chieu: Vietnam's Martial Arts Missionary," CNN, November 26, 2014, http://edition.cnn.com/2014/11/26/sport/human-to-hero-nguyen-van-chieu-vovinam-martial-art-vietnam/index.html.

61 European Vovinam Federation, "Vovinam History," 2014, http://www.vovinam-evvf.eu/evvf/history/.

62 Nguyen Tri, "Vovinam," June 14, 2003, http://atlantamartialarts.com/styles/vovinam.htm.

63 Michael Tran, "Vovinam/Viet Vo Dao", in *Martial Arts of the World: An Encyclopedia*, Edited by Thomas A Green, (Santa Barbara, CA: ABC-CLIO, 2001), 441.

64 Ibid.

65 Knight and Maguder, "Nguyen Van Chieu," CNN, 2014, para. 10.

66 Tran, "Vovinam", in Martial Arts of the World, 655.

67 Bui Tuan Dat, Vovinam Master, in discussion with the author, Cau Lac Bo BTD, Ngo 159, Cau Giay District, Hanoi, March 2016.

68 European Vovinam Federation, "Vovinam Characteristics," 2014, http://www.vovinam-evvf.eu/evvf/ characteristics/, para. 4.

69 Ibid., para. 1.

70 Tran, "Vovinam", in Martial Arts of the World, 655.

71 Mai Anh, "Master Hoang Thanh Phong: Nearly 35 Years of Contributing to Spreading Traditional Martial Arts in Schools," January 28, 2019, http://thethaovietnam.vn/chuyen-the-thao/vo-su-hoang-thanh-phong-gan-35-nam-gop-phan-truyen-ba-vo-thuat-co-truyen-trong-hoc-duong-397-325702.html.

72 Vo Duong Thanh Phong, "Thanh Phong School Introduction," 2019, http://www.voduongthanhphong.com/.

73 Ibid., para. 1.

74 Hoang Thanh Phong, Founder of Thanh Phong School, in discussion with the author, Phan Dinh Phung Street, Hoan Kiem District, Hanoi, September 2015.

75 Ibid.

76 Ibid.

77 Vo Duong Thanh Phong, "Thanh Phong School Introduction".

78 Mai Hac Long, "Võ Việt Nơi Địa Đầu Tổ Quốc," Liên Đoàn Võ Thuật Cổ Truyền Việt Nam, December 1, 2016, http://vocotruyenvietnam.vn/van-hoa-vo-thuat/cac-mon-vo-viet-nam/vo-viet-noi-dia-dau-to-quoc.aspx.

79 Lee, Gary Yia, and Nicholas Tapp, Culture and Customs of the Hmong, (Santa Barbara, CA: Greenwood, 2010), 9.

80 Mai, "Võ Việt Nơi Địa", 2016.

81 Nguyen Thang Long, "Bắc Việt Võ—Công Phu Bí Truyền Vùng Tây Bắc Việt Nam., Người Đưa Tin, September 2, 2017, https://www.nguoiduatin.vn/bac-viet-vo-cong-phu-bi-truyen-vung-tay -bac-viet-nam-a334237.html.

CHAPTER TWO FIGURES

Figure 3.—Nhat Nam Martial Art International. Nhat Nam School Logo, 2010, http://nhat-nam.org/

Figure 4.—Provided by Le Trung Linh, Nam Hong Son School Logo, 2013, https://www.facebook.com/namhongsonquanngua/

Figure 5.—Vovinam—Viet Vo Dao Federation. Vovinam School Logo, June 18, ·2013. Wikimedia Commons. https://commons.wikimedia.org/wiki/File:VVN_logo.jpg.

Figure 6.—Wikimedia Commons, Nguyen Loc. March 18, 2017, Wikimedia Commons. https://commons.wikimedia.org/wiki/File:NguyenLoc.jpg.

Figure 7.—Douglas Pike, Tết Trung Thu 1969—Defense Skills—Douglas Pike Photograph Collection, February 10, 2012. Flickr. https://www.flickr.com/photos/97930879@N02/10849550636.

Figures 8-14.—Provided by Hoang Thanh Phong, September 13, 2015, Flickr. https://www.flickr.com/photos/113413385@N07/30178800707/.

Figure 15. Bac Viet Vo School Logo, 2015, https://www.facebook.com/bacvietvo.

CENTRAL VIETNAMESE STYLES AND SCHOOLS

POINTS OF INTEREST

Laos
Thailand
Cambodia
Vietnam

Hue Province
The Central Highlands
Binh Dinh
Province

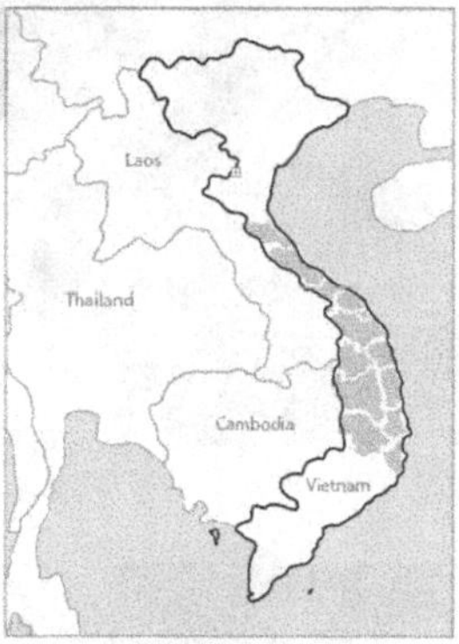

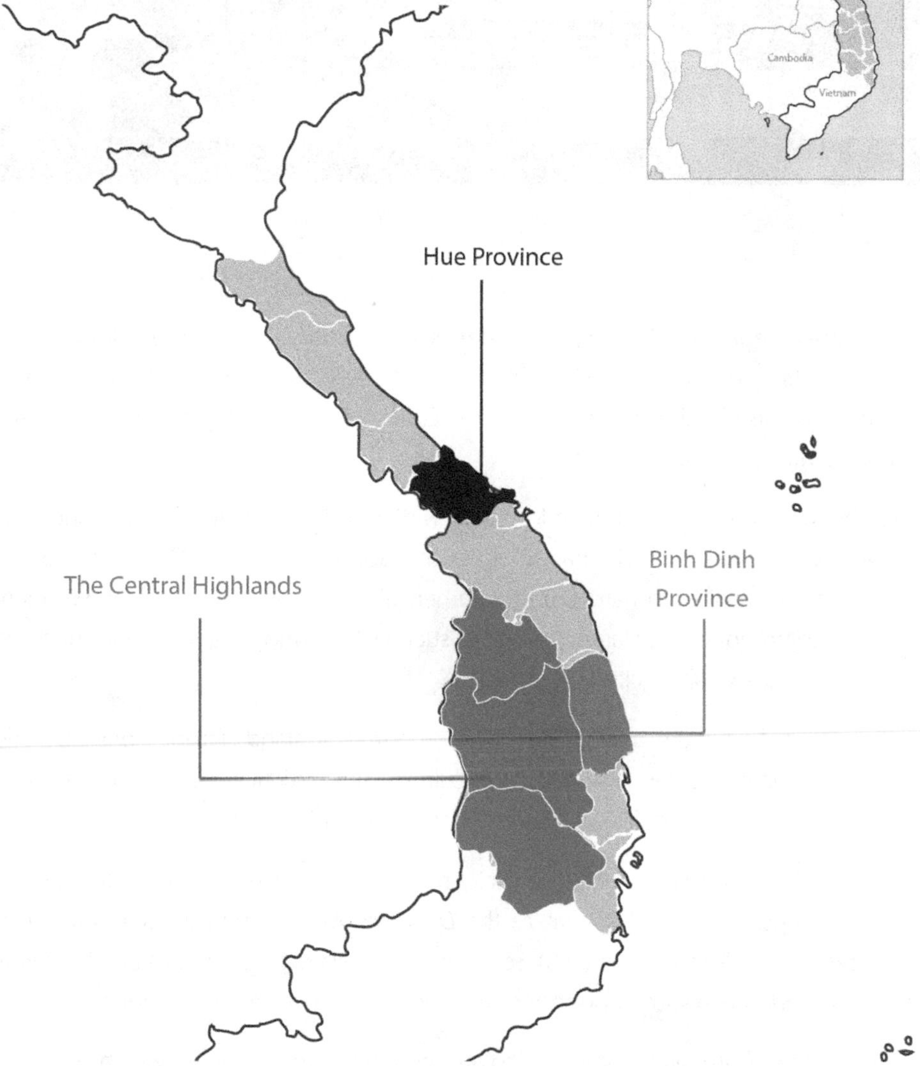

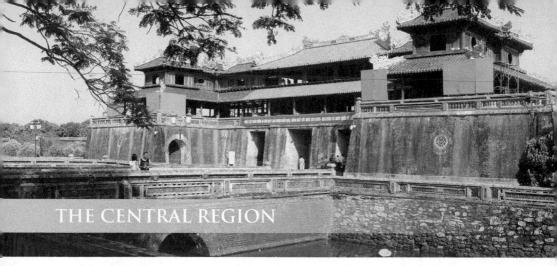

THE CENTRAL REGION

The main gate of the Nguyen Dynasty Citadel in Hue Province

The central region of Vietnam, or **Annam** as it was known during the colonial period, stretches from Thanh Hoa Province in the north to Dak Lak Province in the south-central highlands and Khanh Hoa Province on the coast. In total, the region covers an area of around 140,000 square kilometers.

To the east is a narrow strip of lowlands with hundreds of kilometers of incredible beaches, forests and fields that sit upon the South China Sea. The coastline is an important area of both natural and commercial resources, as it is dotted with small fishing communities and larger port-cities such as Quy Nhon, Da Nang and the former Nguyen Dynasty capital city, Hue.

Inland from the picturesque coastline are the central highlands, famous for their diverse range of wildlife, cooler climate and agriculture—in particular the globally-renowned variety of Vietnamese coffee, as well as tobacco, tea and rubber.

Besides a large population of Viet ethnicity, the central highlands are home to numerous tribal groups, collectively known as the **Degar** or **Montagnard** (meaning **Mountain People** or **Mountaineers** in French). Some of the largest of these groups are the **Bahnar**, **Jarai** and **Ede**, each with populations between two and five hundred thousand.[83]

Toward the south of the central region lies Binh Dinh Province, which is an area considered by many to be synonymous with martial arts.[84]

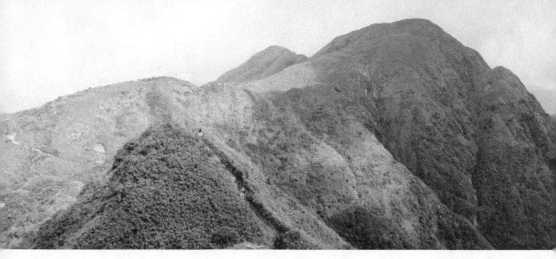

Although the Viet people have only consistently inhabited Binh Dinh Province since the seventeenth century, there are various historical factors for the province's reputation as a martial hotspot.

The provincial capital city of Quy Nhon was the site of the former Champa Kingdom city-state, **Vijaya,** and is dotted with relics of the ancient warrior civilization. Since its founding in the twelfth century, Vijaya was a significant Southeast Asian trading port with the trade winds bringing in ships from the Malay Peninsula, China and across the Indian Ocean.[85]

In more recent times, many followers of the Nguyen Clan, including numerous skilled martial artists settled the region and mixed with Cham and Highland groups. Similarly, during the short but pivotal period of the Tay Son Rebellion (1771 1792) trade routes ran from the port of Quy Nhon into the western highlands, connecting the central provinces to the north and south. Finally, the city of Hue later became the capital of the Nguyen Dynasty, further solidifying the region's martial legacy throughout the nineteenth and twentieth century.

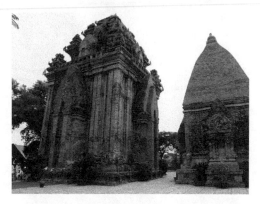

Champa era temples in Nha Trang, Khanh Hoa Province

In this chapter we will look at the modern-day martial arts from the central region of Vietnam. First, we will provide an overview of the umbrella style of **Võ Cổ Truyền**, which is an amalgamated system of various Binh Dinh schools (similar in some respects to the modern Chinese martial art system of Wushu). We will then take a closer look at some of the oldest traditional schools in the region that stem from local family styles, before finally examining the martial arts of the Imperial Guard from the former Vietnamese Nguyen Dynasty capital, Hue.

Binh Dinh Province Martial Arts

(Võ Bình Định / Võ Cổ Truyền / Võ Tây Sơn)

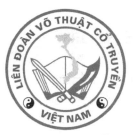

Fig. 16.

The central region of Vietnam is arguably the most important in the development of what we now know as the Vietnamese martial arts. The modern styles stemming from the region are collectively referred to as *Võ Cổ Truyền*, *Võ Bình Định* or *Võ Tây Sơn* (*Traditional Vietnamese Martial Arts/Martial Arts from Binh Dinh Province/Tay Son District*).

Due to a combination of the region's turbulent history, the warrior spirits of its inhabitants and the promotion of Vietnamese martial arts as a source of patriotism and national identity, Vo Co Truyen has a large following both throughout Vietnam and across the globe. The Binh Dinh region martial arts are often considered by Vietnamese scholars to have emerged from the province in a similar manner to how Chinese "Kung Fu," is claimed to have stemmed from a single region and source. However, in the case of Vietnam, a closer look at the history reveals otherwise.

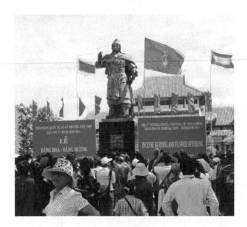

The Quang Trung Temple in An Nhon Village, Binh Dinh Province

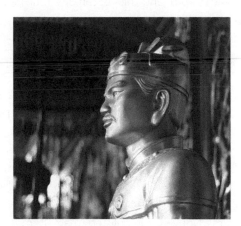

An effigy of Quang Trung upon the main temple altar

HISTORY

The legacy of Binh Dinh region martial arts is likely to have begun with the Cham, who are known to have had important trade routes and significant military presence in Vijaya from at least the tenth century.[87] The Cham people have a long history as warriors and martial arts practices that served both military purposes and religious rituals can be observed in various sculptures and artworks of the Champa Kingdom.[88] However, Cham martial arts are no longer practiced (publicly at least within Vietnam).

The Cham population were famously seafarers, who often traveled from Mainland Southeast Asia throughout the Malay Peninsula and beyond. This may have relevance as certain schools of Malaysian Silat are also known to trace their lineage back to Cham martial art masters.[89] While even the development of some weapons, such as the distinct, curved Southeast Asian sword, the *Kris*, is considered by some scholars to have originated within the Champa Kingdom.[90]

In the highlands on the western border of central Vietnam, groups of the Degar/Montagnard have survived for centuries by honing their agricultural and hunting skills—specializing in the use of weapons such as the machete and crossbow. Throughout these highlands, traditional martial arts, particularly in the form of dance-like performances with swords and shields, can often still be observed, while groups such as the Jarai and Ede are well known for their history of tribal warfare.[91]

From the tenth century onward, Viet Empire to the north began to expand south and gradually assimilated itself into new surroundings and societies. In doing so, the Viet people brought with them the already thousand-year-old practices of the sword and spear, as well as concepts such as traditional wrestling and unarmed battlefield combat. This cross cohabitation of martial cultures peaked with the Nguyen progression southwards in the seventeenth century.

A resurgence of martial arts practices is said to have followed the Tay Son Rebellion, which emerged from Binh Dinh Province during the late Eighteenth century. At this time Nguyen Hue enlisted Cham, Khmer and ethnic Highlanders alongside groups of Chinese and Viet peasants, bandits and pirates for the Tay Son military.

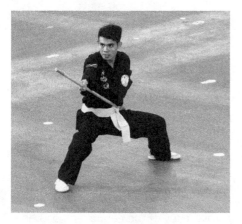
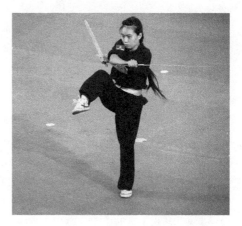

A traditional staff form   *Phoenix Double Sword Form*

Nguyen Hue and his two warrior brothers, Nguyen Nhac and Nguyen Lu, are also widely credited with the creation of several techniques and forms of Vo Co Truyen,[92] while many of the modern-day schools in the region claim direct lineages to the warriors of the Tay Son Rebellion and their teachers, such as Truong Van Hien.

During this period, many Binh Dinh villages developed reputations for producing warriors. Some of the most renowned are Thuan Truyen, An Thai and An Vinh, all of which are well known for their unique and formidable styles. The local population summarizes the village specialties with sayings such as:

"Roi Thuận Truyền, Quyền An Vinh":
"Thuan Truyen village for staffs and An Vinh village for fists."

"Trai An Thái, Gái An Vinh":
"An Thai style for men, An Vinh style for women."[93]

The former of these sayings is said to have arisen due to the strengths of specific martial families, while the latter is because the An Thai style emphasizes strength whereas the An Vinh style emphasizes speed.

Allegedly, the An Thai style martial arts were developed by a second-generation Chinese immigrant named Diep Truong Phat, who found refuge in the region and incorporated aspects of Chinese martial arts into the local system to create a particularly effective style.[94] In contrast, An Vinh Village was said to have been founded by Nguyen

Ngac, a female descendant of Bui Thi Xuan, one of the most skilled female warriors of the Tay Son Dynasty and creator of a double-sword fighting style which is thought to have attributed to her successes as a general.[95]

In the nineteenth century, local martial arts systems grew in popularity. They were openly trained by the Imperial Guard and public examinations were held in the new capital city of Hue. Meanwhile, much of the Cham culture was abolished by Emperor Minh Mang who ordered the dismantling of a Cham protectorate, outlawed many Hindu and Islam practices and decreed that indigenous Cham and Khmer people were required "to dress like the Vietnamese, eat like the Vietnamese, and learn Vietnamese."[96] This process of Vietnamization was repeated across many of the central and southern provinces in attempts to forge national identity, which in turn led to a great deal of ambiguity regarding martial arts practices and the ethnic backgrounds of various important figures in their development.[97]

Nowadays, Vo Co Truyen schools are found all across Vietnam and are prominently displayed during festivals and New Year celebrations—Lion Dances and weapon forms are often performed in a nod to Vietnam's military history.

The governing body of traditional martial arts (the Vo Co Truyen Association of Vietnam) is active in promoting the system, while collaboration with equivalent organizations in other countries has led to the development of the International Vietnamese Martial Arts Festival (held in Quy Nhon city every two years). This is a huge event amalgamating traditional Vietnamese martial arts clubs from over sixty countries who come to meet, exchange skills, compete and perform in the homeland of their styles.

Although there are no documented formal training systems of the Highland groups or Cham martial arts continuing in Vietnam, it may be considered that their influences have impacted the development of modern Binh Dinh styles. Meanwhile, there may well be methods of combat training still taking place behind closed doors.

CHARACTERISTICS

Despite influence from various sources and many schools falling under the umbrella term of Vo Co Truyen, there are a number of uniform practices within these styles. They are widely acknowledged to be:

- Physical conditioning. This can take the shape of general fitness training; external "hard" conditioning drills that develop the strength of the bones, muscles and skin through repeated controlled blows; or internal "soft" training practices such as *Qigong* which can be considered as methods for cultivating and directing energy.[98]

- *Bài Quyền (*or *forms)*—set patterns of attacking and defensive movements. These are also broken down into practical applications and drills, with a focus on automating reactions for self-defense purposes.

- Competitive fighting and sparring.

- Weapons training.

While the specific physical conditioning practices may vary between individual styles and instructors, the three latter characteristics have been developed into uniform systems through the collaboration of schools and associations. Each of which is considered in more detail in the following pages.

Competitive fighting

The official regulations for competitive Vo Co Truyen detail a standardized system of full-contact competition. Within this rule set, practitioners wear 12-14 oz gloves, headgear and chest protectors—similar to the attire of Taekwondo or Sport Karate, and they are awarded points for the accurate execution of techniques.[99]

Unlike many modern ring-sports, sweeps, trips and takedowns are permitted and earn points. However, ground confrontations are disallowed.

Fights feature three rounds of three-minute-long bouts with one-minute rest periods. The winner is the first to defeat his opponent in two out of three rounds—points are awarded for clear hits and takedowns—or by knockout/technical knockout.

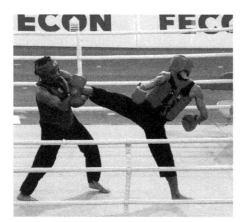 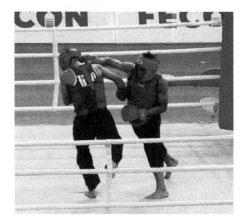

A kick followed by a hard punch in combination with a foot sweep won the round

FORMS

Grandmaster Truong Van Vinh, summarizes the mantra of Vo Co Truyen as *"**Nhanh, Mạnh, Chính Xác**,"* meaning *"**Speed, Strength and Accuracy**."*[100] According to Vinh, these skills do not come quickly, but must be developed over time and through repetition. This is something that can be achieved through the practice of forms or *Bài Quyền*, which are central to the style.

Within Vo Co Truyen, each form is considered to teach a fundamental skill set for a specific fighting style, as a result, a single form/style may take many years of practice to perfect. Advanced forms feature an array of weapons, empty-handed and animal styles; they are often memorized through poems that describe their movements and theory, many of which can be traced back to the early settlers of Binh Dinh Province.[101]

These poems serve as both step-by-step instructions and provide students with a better understanding of the philosophy behind the style. An example is the form of *Tứ Linh Đao*, which is described in an eighteen-line poem, an extract follows:

'Hướng Đông chấp thủ nghiêm chào
Chụm về tay phải cầm đao loan liền
Lui chân, tay kéo lên trên
Chém qua trái, phải, vớt liền một phen
Nghiêng về rùa núp lá sen
Chém ngang phát cỏ, bay lên Phượng Hoàng'

"Turn to the east, attention and salute,
The right hand grasps the broadsword,
Step backward, the hand pulls the sword up,
Left cut, right cut and uppercut in a single motion,
Sloping back like a turtle hiding behind lotus,
Slashing horizontally, then rise up like Phoenix"[102]

Although the forms/styles practiced by individual schools vary based upon instructor preferences and specialties, ten of the key forms of Vo Co Truyen include:

- *"Bát Quái Côn—Eight Trigram Staff Form*
- *Độc Lư Thương—Poison Spear Form*
- *Hùng Kê Quyền—Golden Rooster Form*
- *Huỳnh Long Độc Kiếm—Poison Dragon Sword Form*
- *Lão Hổ Thượng Sơn—Wise Tiger Ascending the Mountain*
- *Lão Mai Quyền—Plum Blossom Form*
- *Ngọc Trản Quyền—Jade Jewel Form*
- *Roi Thái Sơn—Thai Son Staff Form*
- *Siêu Xung Thiên—Halberd Form*
- *Tứ Linh Đao—Four Spirit Animal Swords."*[103]

Many forms of Vo Co Truyen have interesting backstories that tie into the history and traditions of the region, specifically *Hùng Kê Quyền* and *Độc Lư Thương* which are said to have been devised by Nguyen Lu and Nguyen Nhac, respectively.[104]

In modern practices, links like these to historical warriors and battlefield practices are viewed favorably; they are often seen as evidence of effectiveness or factors that add legitimacy to their practices. These forms are detailed below.

HÙNG KÊ QUYỀN

Hùng Kê Quyền or *The Golden Rooster Form* imitates the moves of the animal in battle (cock fighting is widely practiced in Southeast Asian culture). The origins of the form are said to come from the youngest brother of Quang Trung, Nguyen Lu—who was sent to oversee the southern forces following the Tay Son Rebellion. It is said that Nguyen Lu wanted to develop a precise martial arts program for his military units but knew that training in traditional styles was too time-consuming and impractical for the rate of development his army required.[105]

While attending a cock fight during Lunar New Year celebrations, Nguyen Lu observed that, time after time, the smaller cock would attack the large, proud rooster he was pitted against with vicious strikes, kicking, scratching and pecking at its eyes—as a result the vicious, smaller cock won. Nguyen Lu, being of a small stature, compared both himself and the Viet people to the smaller rooster and decided that they needed this kind of precise aggression to be successful in battle. According to Ngo Bong, one of the top masters of the Golden Rooster Style, the newly-developed form was soon implemented among Nguyen Lu's soldiers with ease and is considered to have helped with his further domination of the south.[106]

Inspired by the movements of the cock, Hung Ke Quyen features low kicks to the knees and ankle joints, scratching and tearing at the eyes and sharp precise stabs at vital pressure-points through lateral angles of attack.[107] These movements were designed to inflict maximum damage while remaining possible to perform when dressed in battle armor; consequently, aesthetically satisfying movements were abandoned for those which were more brutal and battle effective.

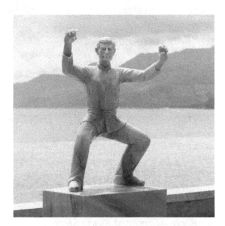

A statue depicting Hung Ke Quyen on Quy Nhon beachfront

ĐỘC LU THUONG

This form translates as **Poison Spear** and is said to have originated in the western highlands (modern-day An Khe, Gia Lai Province), when the three brothers of the Tay Son Rebellion: Quang Trung, Nguyen Nhac and Nguyen Lu worked together. [108]

The three conquered the region quickly during 1770, and as battle-hardened warriors who were skilled in the use of swords and spears, they made a collective effort to devise their own weaponized fighting system.

One of the products of their labor was **Độc Lư Thương**, a spear form which allowed entire garrisons of the brothers' forces to be trained in a uniform battlefield style—thus the form is considered by modern practitioners to represent unity. **Độc Lư Thương** contains forty-one moves and uses a **Giáo** (a six-foot-long spear with a foot-long tip) to thrust and stab with explosive speed.

Weapons

Historically, more than forty types of weapons are thought to have been associated with Vo Co Truyen, however modern practices usually incorporate a standard set of eighteen.[109] These include both typical Southeast Asian weapons and tools, such as axes and machetes, as well those which are more commonly associated with the northern (Chinese) battlefield martial arts, such as broadswords, halberds and spears. The eighteen standard weapons follow.

- **"Bừa Cào**—*Rake*
- **Côn Roi**—*Long Staff*
- **Cung Tên**—*Bow and Arrow*
- **Đao**—*Sword, includes: the* **Đơn Đao** *(Broadsword) and* **Đại Đao** *(Halberd)*
- **Đinh Ba**—*Pitchfork/Tiger Fork*
- **Giản (Thiết Lĩnh)**—*Scepter*
- **Giáo**—*Wide-Tipped Spear*
- **Kích**—*Crescent Blade Staff*
- **Kiếm**—*Straight Sword*
- **Lăng Khiên**—*Shield with Broad Sword*
- **Song Câu**—*Dual Hook Swords*
- **Song Chùy**—*Dual Maces*
- **Song Tô**—*Dual Machetes*
- **Song Phủ Và Búa**—*Dual Axes (or Axe and Hammer)*
- **Song Xỉ**—*Dual Forearm Blades*
- **Thương**—*Pointed Spear*
- **Xà Mâu**—*Serpent Spear*
- **Xích**—*Chain Whip"*[110]

Uniforms

The uniforms of Vo Co Truyen usually consist of black, long-sleeved, button-up shirts and black pants, emblazoned with a particular school or lineage logo.

Students also wear a sash that indicates rank. Beginners wear black sashes and as their skill improves they progress to lighter colors; blue, red, yellow and finally to white, which is said to represent purity, infinity and spirit. Masters wear white sashes, adorned with red or gold stripes indicating their level of mastery.

Benefits of Vo Co Truyen Training

- Accessibility: With a unified governing body, branches throughout the globe and a number of online and in-print learning resources available, Vo Co Truyen is one of the most easily-found styles of Vietnamese martial arts, both in Vietnam and internationally.

- Variety: Vo Co Truyen features everything from full-combat sport fighting to traditional weapons and mediation, ensuring there is something within the system for everyone.

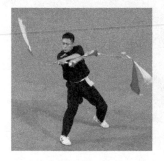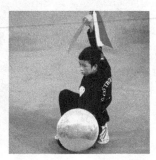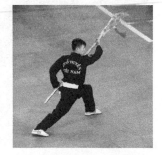

Students demonstrate the weapons Chain Whip, Sword and Shield and Halberd

THE TRADITIONAL SCHOOLS
OF BINH DINH PROVINCE

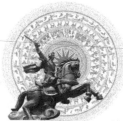

Fig. 17.

This section will examine four famous traditional martial arts schools located within the Tay Son area of Binh Dinh Province.

There are hundreds of schools in the region, therefore the following in no way constitutes a comprehensive list but provides examples of those practices widely recognized for their authenticity or historical lineages.

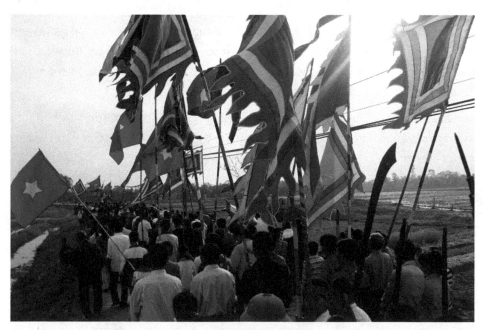

The opening parade of a traditional martial arts festival

LY TUONG MARTIAL ARTS SCHOOL

VÕ ĐƯỜNG LÝ TƯỜNG

Grandmaster Ly Xuan Hy—the former Vice-President of the Binh Dinh Martial Arts Association and founder of the Ly Tuong School—is regarded as an elder of the local martial arts community. His school is widely known for the skill and quantity of martial arts students they produce.

HISTORY

Ly Xuan Hy was born in a rural area in the north of Binh Dinh Province in 1940 and from a young age was taught martial arts by his father and grandfather—the Patriarch Master of the style—known as Ly Tuong.

Ly Tuong famously developed his own martial art forms based upon a mixture of his previous studies and the motions of a cat he had observed skillfully evading capture. He then taught these forms to his sons and grandsons.

Grandmaster Ly Xuan Hy, following the teachings of his Grandfather, was obsessed with martial arts and, from the age of eighteen to thirty-five, traveled through much of the country fighting competitively in full-contact competitions and exchanges. Ly claims that during these years he fought over three hundred matches and lost only once to a master from Saigon in the 1970s. He then went on to research further and receive training from the victor to incorporate into his own style.[111]

From the 1980s onwards Grandmaster Ly has continued to practice and teach in his ancestral village. The school is now run by his son Ly Xuan Van, who teaches throughout Binh Dinh Province and the rest of Vietnam, as well as having branches in several European countries.[112]

Characteristics

Although the Ly Tuong martial arts school includes many standard Vo Co Truyen practices in their syllabus, the defining feature of their system is the form of *Miêu Tẩy Diện* or *The Cat Washing its Face*.

The form comprises of twenty moves that imitate cat-like movements, however, unlike common Tiger or Leopard-style martial arts, Ly Tuong's cat is calm and evasive rather than aggressive.

The Cat Washing its Face refers to use of the paws (hands) circling or covering the head, giving the practitioner a constant defense. In addition to clawing and scratching movements, the forms feature light-footed and quick, evasive maneuvers to resemble a cat dodging and weaving.[113]

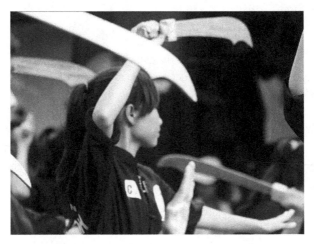

Young students practicing in Tuy Phuoc Village, Binh Dinh Province

Long Phuoc Pagoda Martial Arts

VÕ ĐƯỜNG CHÙA LONG PHƯỚC

Chùa Long Phước is a famous pagoda in Tuy Phuoc District, Binh Dinh Province. Due to its history as both a renowned holy and martial arts site, the pagoda receives thousands of visitors annually and is one of the region's top destinations for visiting martial artists.

History

Due to the methodical preservation of official documentation, the history of Long Phuoc Pagoda is well resourced and there is an extensive archive of antique books that detail the region's martial arts from the time of the Le Dynasty to the Tay Son Dynasty (1428–1802).

According to school manuscripts, a wandering monk named Hu Minh passed through Binh Dinh Province in 1571. He felt a connection with the region and chose to settle at the nearby mountain of Phuoc Thuan, over the years he then built up Long Phuoc Pagoda. Hu Minh researched, preserved and collected famous local martial arts routines; he added various features to create a new system for the monks in the pagoda.

These martial arts were designed to keep the monks' minds and bodies sharp and to offer protection for their order in otherwise turbulent times. From 1571 to the modern day, martial arts have been passed down through the monastic lineage for thirteen generations.[114]

Over the years, not only pagoda residents, but disciples from far and wide have visited the pagoda to pay homage to the monks

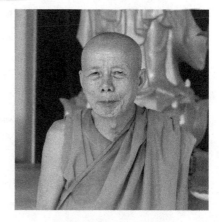

A senior monk of Long Phuoc Pagoda

and study their martial arts. Traditionally, the masters of the pagoda taught only their disciples; however, since 1986 Long Phuoc Pagoda has become more progressive and openly teaches classes to members of the public.

According to Abbot Thich Hanh Hoa, the teaching of the Long Phuoc style is carried out to preserve the spirit of traditional Binh Dinh region martial arts and spread the word of the Buddha. Students learn to follow the Buddhist code of only using violence as a last resort and train for the purpose of spiritual and physical well-being. The motto of the school is *"Bi, Trí, Dũng Của Nhà Phật,"* which translates as *"Compassion, Wisdom and Courage of the Buddha."*[115]

The Nuns of the pagoda also continue to embody both the spirit of Buddhism and of the region's famous female fighters by teaching classes to raise money for local charities, such as for those who have birth defects resulting from the use of Agent Orange during the second Indochina War.

Due in part to their decision to open their doors to the public more than thirty years ago, Long Phuoc Pagoda has been officially identified as a cultural heritage site by the Sports and Culture Department of Binh Dinh Province. Many Buddhist and martial arts disciples make pilgrimages to Long Phuoc Pagoda each year for training and events, exemplifying the importance of the site as a hotspot for religious, historical and martial arts activities.

Characteristics

The Long Phuoc Pagoda school teaches a diverse system that incorporates a range of weapons as well as unarmed methods. However, they are particularly renowned for staff fighting. Historically, sticks were often seen more favorably than other weapons by the Buddhist clergy. This is due to the fact that they were both easily accessible for the monks within their daily lives and were a weapon that could be used in a variety of non-lethal contexts, while attacking somebody with a sword nearly always carries the intent of causing death (one of the worst acts possible for a follower of Buddhism).[116]

Unlike the black attire worn by students of many of the local martial arts schools, members of the Buddhist congregation of Long Phuoc Pagoda are easily recognizable by their light brown robes—the everyday color of Vietnamese Buddhists and lay-initiated practitioners.

PHI LONG VINH MARTIAL ARTS SCHOOL

VÕ ĐƯỜNG PHI LONG VỊNH

The Phi Long Vinh Martial Arts School is one of the best-known institutions of Binh Dinh Province. Their reputation has been earned in part by Grandmaster Truong Van Vinh, who is somewhat of a modern-day martial arts legend. The modest Phi Long Vinh School headquarters are based in Phuoc Son Hamlet, Tuy Phuoc District, Binh Dinh Province.

HISTORY

Grandmaster Vinh states that his family style officially began with his great, great, grandfather, the legendary martial artist named Master Truong Van Hien who taught both martial arts and philosophy to the three Tay Son Rebellion brothers Quang Trung, Nguyen Nhac and Nguyen Lu. In addition to training the famous warriors, Master Hien was said to have continued teaching his children and grandchildren, who subsequently kept the style alive. The modern incarnation of the Phi Long Vinh school was founded by the great-grandfather of Truong Van Vinh in the nineteenth century, it was then led by his father Truong Van Can who reluctantly had to give up teaching as he approached his ninetieth decade.[117]

The Phi Long Vinh School is currently headed by Grandmaster Vinh along with multiple instructors—including his sons—who are settled throughout Binh Dinh and the central provinces. According to Vinh, he is particularly proud of the thousands of high-quality students his school has produced and to have introduced his family style to multiple countries throughout Asia and Europe.[118]

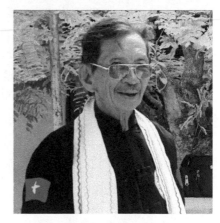

Grandmaster Truong Van Vinh at Long Phuoc Pagoda in 2014

Characteristics

Although the Phi Long Vinh School teach many different elements of martial arts, they are best known for *Ngọc Trản Quyền* (*Jade Bowl Form*) and the historical ties through their family lineage to Quang Trung and the masters before him.

The *Ngọc Trản Quyền* form can be traced back to the original texts of the Truong Clan and it features a routine of twenty-eight techniques that emphasize a combination of soft and hard movements.[119] Practitioners of Ngoc Tran Quyen learn to attack with both aggression and force as well as use the attacker's own strength against them through rotating stances and evasive techniques in a similar manner to Tai Chi or Aikido. The ability to switch rapidly between these defensive and offensive aspects is one of the key features of the form.

Vinh considers his family style to have been shaped significantly by both its origins in the agricultural lowlands of Binh Dinh Province and the prohibition of training for many years. As a result, the system incorporates many low stances, throws and sweeps; which may have developed from practitioners needing to defend themselves against soldiers, while keeping clear of sword or spear stabbing range. Similarly, the rural roots of the style that supported a rebellion of peasants and marginalized peoples can be seen in the many traditional farming implements that are used as weaponry, including hoes, shovels, sticks and staffs.

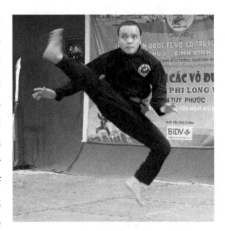

A Phi Long Vinh School Student demonstrating a form

LE XUAN CANH SCHOOL

VÕ ĐƯỜNG LÊ XUÂN CẢNH

A style of Vo Co Truyen renowned for their weapon skills, is that of Grandmaster Le Xuan Canh and his self-titled school. The Le Xuan Canh School is said to focus on developing the spirit and art of training through sharing knowledge and inclusive (often free) tuition.[120]

HISTORY

Le Xuan Canh was born in 1938 in Cam Van Village, An Nhon District. He studied martial arts from the age of fifteen and after a year of intensive study under Master Ly Tuong, he decided to travel around the province and collect more techniques from famed schools in An Nhon and Tuy Phuoc District.

Although Xuan Canh rarely competed in martial arts contests or openly displayed his abilities, word of his skill soon traveled and he decided to begin accepting students. In 1975, the Le Xuan Canh School officially opened its doors to students and soon became recognized for their performances in contests and competitions both across Vietnam and internationally, earning particular respect for flawless performances with weapon forms.

Grandmaster Le Xuan Canh still accepts and trains students in Cam Van Village, An Nhon Province, often asking only for donations from students rather than fees.[121]

CHARACTERISTICS

The Le Xuan Canh School is highly regarded throughout the province for their blended system of local Binh Dinh family styles. Dual-weapon techniques, such as double-sword forms, are considered as one of the specialties of the school. Other standout aspects are the training of "soft" weapons such as whips, scarves and belts which can be utilized to tie up and subdue opponents. This is said to have particular efficiency when used against those armed with "hard" weapons such as swords or staffs.[122]

The Le Xuan Canh School has also been prominent in keeping traditional martial arts performances alive. Students of the school train in Lion Dance to a high level and are one of the few groups to continue the practice of "Human Chess" in which skilled martial artists take up roles as Chinese Chess pieces and stage mock-battles as moves take place. Both of these practices are commonly held as performances over festivals during the Vietnamese Lunar New Year.

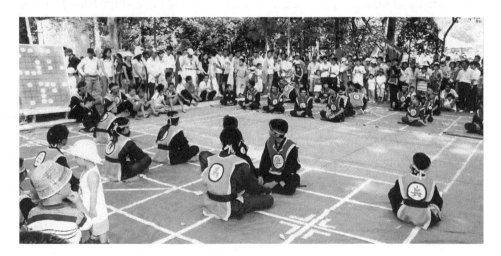

Fig. 18. Students dressed as chess pieces waiting for their "turn" to play during a festival in Ho Chi Minh City

VAN AN PHAI SCHOOL

VÕ KINH VẠN AN PHÁI

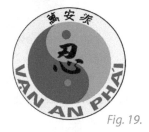

Fig. 19.

The Van An Phai School of martial arts is based in the central province and former capital city of the Nguyen Dynasty, Hue. The name *Võ Kinh Vạn An Phái* literally translates as *The Vietnamese Way of Infinite Peace/Security*.

History

According to masters of the Van An Phai School, the first incarnation of the modern system was developed by a military commander named Nguyen Huu Canh under the order of the Emperor Nguyen Anh (Gia Long) who ruled the nation from 1802–1820.[123]

During the relatively recent, yet turbulent Nguyen Dynasty which lasted up until 1945, soldiers protecting the royal family and capital city were required to have the skills both to defend Hue from potential attacks and to maintain control and order among the civilian population. As a result, a number of Binh Dinh region martial arts were adapted and refined into a system of self-defense and physical training for the Imperial Guard.

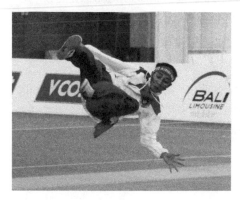
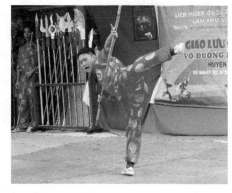

Vo Kinh Van An Phai students demonstrate flying kicks and a staff form

Following the collapse of the Vietnamese feudal system—brought about by the abdication of the throne by Emperor Bao Dai in 1945—many martial arts, including the Van An Phai School, were outlawed. However, several former-Imperial-Guard masters are thought to have kept the practices alive by training and teaching their martial arts skills in secret.[124]

The Van An Phai School was founded by Master Truong Van Thang who started teaching formally (albeit in secrecy) in 1945 before officially opening his school to the public in 1972. Truong Van Thang was a disciple of Grandmaster Nguyen Thanh Van, who himself was trained by the Imperial Guard and appointed officially as Grandmaster by the Nguyen regime.[125]

The Van An Phai School is currently headed by Master Truong Quang Kim, the son of Truong Van Thang and the fifth generation of Van An Phai masters. Since 2000, Kim has successfully spread the tradition to a number of countries, including France, the United States, Italy and Australia. The school maintains its headquarters in the ancient capital city of Hue and offers training to Vietnamese and foreign students alike. They also feature a specialized program for underprivileged local children, this is supported by income earned from exhibitions and cultural performances that can often be seen in and around Hue.

CHARACTERISTICS

The Van An Phai School incorporates many different features into its syllabus. While physical techniques are trained at all levels, high-ranking students are also expected to study theory, *Qigong* and traditional medicine alongside combatives in a similar manner to the examinations of the Nguyen Dynasty Imperial Guard.[126]

One of the unique aspects of this style is its focus on self-defense and conflict resolution. Students often learn a number of immobilization techniques and non-lethal civilian weapons, alongside those more suited for the battlefield, a feature that may have been incorporated due to its use as a training and peacekeeping tool of the Imperial Guard.

Besides weapons, the Van An Phai style features a number of highly-dynamic and acrobatic forms. Many of the forms are based upon common martial arts animals, including the Tiger, Leopard, Monkey, Snake, Eagle and Dragon, while others are more typically Vietnamese, such as the Cat and Buffalo.[127]

Although training uniforms vary across individual clubs, students often practice in a simple black long-sleeved shirt and pants. Public performances may also incorporate traditional Imperial Guard outfits, such as an *Áo Dài*—literally meaning **Long Shirt** or **Robe**—made of gold and red silk, with a Vietnamese conical hat.

The *Áo Dài* is the national dress of Vietnam. Although it remains popular attire for women, it is generally worn by men only during special occasions.

Benefits of Van An Phai training

- Cardiovascular fitness: Due to the dynamic and explosive style of Van An Phai form practices, a high level of fitness is emphasized among practitioners.

- Practicality: The modern peacekeeping and self-defense aspects of the system provide a martial art which may appear better suited for modern life than other traditional equivalents.

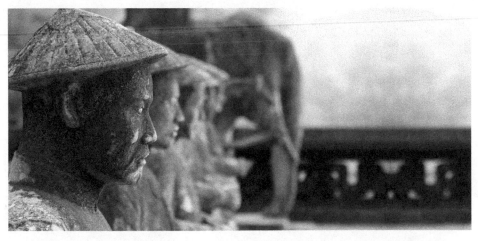

The "Imperial Guard" lined up at the tomb of the Nguyen Kings on the outskirts of Hue

CHAPTER THREE NOTES

[83] Nguyen, Van Huy, Dai Duy Le, Thao Quy Nguyen, and Thao Xuan Vu, *Đại Gia Đình Các Dân Tộc Việt Nam: The Great Family of Ethnic Groups in Vietnam*, (Hanoi: Giáo Dục Publishers), 2014.

[84] Ngoc Huu and Lady Borton, *Martial Arts—Võ Dân Tộc*, (Hanoi, Thế Giới Publishers, 2005), 31.

[85] Goscha, Christopher E., *The Penguin History of Modern Vietnam*, (London: Penguin Books 2017), 480-483.

[86] Green, Thomas A., *Martial Arts of the World: An Encyclopedia*, (Santa Barbara, CA: ABC-CLIO, 2001), 778.

[87] Taylor, K W., *A History of the Vietnamese*, (Cambridge: Cambridge University Press, 2013).

[88] Ngoc and Borton, *Martial Arts*, 31.

[89] Ismail, Abdul Rahman Haji, *Seni Silat Melayu*, (Kuala Lumpur: Dewan Bahasa dan Pustaka, 2009).

[90] Farish A Noor, "From Majapahit to Putrajaya: The Kris as a Symptom of Civilizational Development and Decline," *South East Asia Research 8*, no. 3 (November 1, 2000): 239–79, https://doi.org/10.5367/000000000101297280.

[91] Phạm Phong, *Lịch Sử Võ Học Việt Nam*, (Ho Chi Minh City: Nhà Xuất Bản Văn Hóa Thông Tin, 2013).

[92] Thuc Giap, "Năm Gà Kể Chuyện Hùng Kê Quyền," January 23, 2005, http://baobinhdinh.com.vn/642/2005/1/18249/.

[93] Phạm, *Lịch Sử Võ*, 238.

[94] Bao Binh Dinh, "Vài Nét Về Bình Thái Đạo," February 11, 2007, http://www.baobinhdinh.com.vn/vemiendatvo/2007/3/40287/, para. 2.

[95] Bao Binh Dinh, "Quyền An Vinh," November 1, 2006, http://www.baobinhdinh.com.vn/vungdatvo/2006/11/34594/.

[96] Goscha, *The Penguin History*, 490.

[97] Thich, Quang Huyen, *Dharma Mountain Buddhism & Martial Yoga*, (Frederick, MD: Dharma Mountain Publications, Chùa Xá Lợi 2010).

[98] Green, *Martial Arts of the World*, 335.

[99] Nguyen Thai Dang, "Về Việc Ban Hành Luật Thi Đấu Võ Cổ Truyền Việt Nam," 2002, https://thuvienphapluat.vn/van-ban/The-thao-Y-te/Quyet-dinh-771-QD- UBTDTT-Luat-thi-dau-Vo-co-truyen- Viet-Nam-93667.aspx.

[100] Truong Van Vinh, Grandmaster Phi Long Vinh School, in discussion with the author, Long Phuoc Pagoda, Tuy Phuoc District, Binh Dinh Province, September 2014.

[101] Phạm, *Lịch Sử Võ*, 598-600.

[102] Vo Thuat, "Bài Quyền Tứ Linh Đao," June 18, 2015, http://www.vothuat. vn/goc-luyen-cong /tuyet-ky-goc-luyen-cong/vo-co-truyen-bai-quyen-tu-linh-dao.html.

[103] Vo Co Truyen Association of Vietnam, "Huỳnh Long Độc Kiếm—10 Bài Quyền Chuẩn Hóa Võ Cổ Truyền Việt Nam," YouTube video, 4:11, December 28, 2018, https://www.youtube.com/watch?v=kulE5H7zjaM.

[104] Thuc Giap, "Năm Gà Kể Chuyện Hùng Kê Quyền," January 23, 2005, http://baobinhdinh.com.vn/642/2005/1/18249/.

[105] Ibid.

[106] Ibid.

[107] Green, *Martial Arts of the World*, 549.

[108] Vo Thuat, "Độc Lư Thương," June 24, 2015, http://www.vothuat.vn/goc-luyen-cong/tu-luyen-vo-thuat/vo-co-truyen-viet-nam-doc-lu-thuong.html.

[109] Phạm, *Lịch Sử Võ*.

[110] Truong Van Bao, "Lược Khảo Binh Khí Võ Cổ Truyền," Liên đoàn võ thuật cổ truyền Việt Nam, August 11, 2015, http://vocotruyenvietnam.vn/van-hoa-vo-thuat/thuat-ngu-vo/luoc-khao-binh-khi-vo-co-truyen.aspx.

[111] Thanh Hai, "Tuyệt Chiêu 'Miêu Tẩy Diện' Bất Bại Của 'Hùm Xám Tây Nguyên,'" Võ Thuật, February 19, 2019, http://www.vothuat.vn/cac-mon-phai/vo-co-truyen/tuyet-chieu-mieu-tay-dien-bat-bai-cua-hum-xam-tay-nguyen.html.

[112] Ibid.

[113] Tinh Hoa Vo Thuat, "Võ Sư Lý Xuân Hỷ—Bộ Chỏ Quyền Miêu Tẩy Diện., VTV4, September 6, 2016, https://www.youtube.com/watch?v=mQr13BkeBx4.

[114] Dang Viet Hong, "Làng Võ Sông Côn - Tập 2 - Tinh Hoa Đất Võ," Truyen Hinh An Vien, January 3, 2014, https://www.youtube.com/watch?v=JRe2uFDao0c.

[115] Ibid., 22:28.

[116] Truong, in discussion with the author, 2014.

[117] Ibid.

[118] Nguyen Ngoc Van, "Một Số Võ Đường Là Điểm Tham Quan Liên Hoan Quốc Tế Võ Cổ Truyền," Bao Binh Dinh, July 27, 2010, http://www.baobinhdinh.com.vn/vemiendatvo/2010/7/94998/.

[119] Phạm, Lịch Sử Võ, 598-600.

[120] Dang, "Làng Võ Sông Côn".

[121] Duong Kha, "Tiên Ông' Làng Võ Bình Định Và Bí Kíp 'Binh Khí' Khăn," Công Lý & Xã Hội, January 29, 2018, https://conglyxahoi.net.vn/phong-su/tien-ong-lang-vo-binh-dinh -va-bi-kip-binh-khi-khan- 9943.html.

[122] Ibid., para. 11-12.

[123] Dinh Phu, "Võ Kinh Vạn An Phái," Thanh Nhien, October 7, 2010, https://thanhnien.vn/doi-song /vo-kinh-van-an-phai -153435.html.

[124] Ibid.

[125] Van An Phai France, "Van An Phai in Viet Nam," 2014, https://www.vananphai.fr/presentation/ van-an-phai-au-viet-nam/.

[126] Loc Thai, "Đặc Sản' Võ Kinh," Tuổi Trẻ, September 19, 2015, https://tuoitre.vn/dac-san-vo-kinh- 971643.htm.

[127] Van An Phai France, "Empty-Handed Practice," 2014, https://www.vananphai.fr/kung-fu-vietnamien/ pratique-a-mains-nues/.

CHAPTER THREE FIGURES

Figure 16.—Lien Doan Vo Co Truyen Vietnam. Vietnamese Traditional Martial Arts Federation Logo, 2014, http://vocotruyenvietnam.vn/default.aspx.

Figure 17.—Binh Dinh Tourism Board, 4th International Festival of Traditional Martial Arts, August 04, 2014, http://lhqtvct.binhdinh.gov.vn/index.php?lang=vi

Figure 18.—Ho Tuong, Một hình thức biểu diễn khá độc đáo của Lớp Võ Lâm Do Võ Sư Hồ Tường truyền dạy ở Nhà Văn Hóa Thanh Niên là Thi đấu biểu diễn Cờ Người Võ Thuật với sự Tham Gia của tất cả võ Sư, huấn luyện Viên và võ Sinh, April 8, 2011, Flickr. https://www.flickr.com/photos/86460686@N02/7944696296/.

Figure 19.—Vo Kinh Van An Phai Organization, Van An Phai School Logo, 2010, https://vo-kinh-van-an-royal-martial-art.business.site/

SOUTH VIETNAMESE STYLES AND SCHOOLS

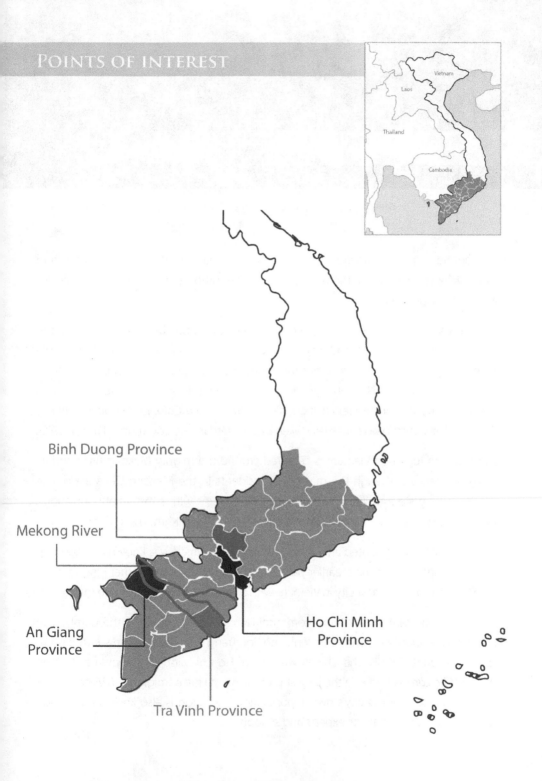

Binh Duong Province

Mekong River

An Giang
Province

Tra Vinh Province

Ho Chi Minh
Province

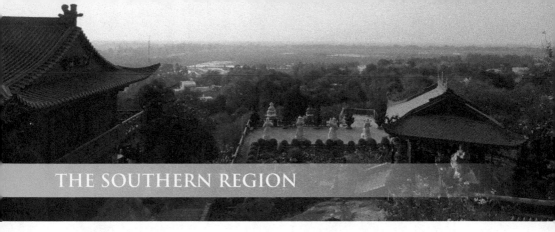

THE SOUTHERN REGION

The Mekong Delta floodplains viewed from the foot of the Seven Mountains

Accounting for roughly a third of the nation's total area—around thirty-nine thousand square kilometers—the southern region of Vietnam is home to a population of almost eighteen million inhabitants.

For many years prior to Viet occupation, much of the south belonged to the Khmer Kingdom. From the seventeenth century, the southern provinces shifted between rule from the Nguyen Dynasty, the Khmer, the Cham or other indigenous groups. Then, from 1862-1954, under the Nguyen Dynasty and the French Colonialists, these provinces became a subdivision of French Indochina known as *La Colonie de Cochinchine* or *Cochinchina*. Control was eventually taken by the Vietnamese Communist Party in 1975.

The southern region of Vietnam is centered around the mighty Mekong River and its many tributaries. Although the majority of residents in the Mekong Delta are of Viet ethnicity, there are a multiplicity of other ethnic groups with substantial populations, such as the Hoa (ethnic Chinese), Khmer Krom (Vietnamese-Khmer) and Cham.

The most-densely populated area is Ho Chi Minh City, which was known as Saigon up until 1976, and *Prey Nokor* in earlier years when it was part of the Khmer Kingdom. Ho Chi Minh is also the largest city in Vietnam with a population of almost nine million.

The most significant Khmer Krom communities can be found along the Cambodian border to the southwest and in Tra Vinh and Soc Trang Provinces on the south-eastern tip of the country. While the Chinatown area of Ho Chi Minh City, known as Cholon District (*Chợ Lớn*), is home to the largest proportion of Hoa immigrants in Vietnam, just over four percent of the city's overall population.[128] Cholon is also known for its high concentration of martial arts experts and schools.

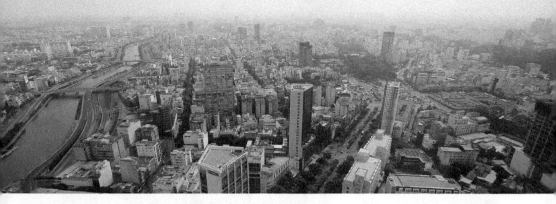

The view of downtown Ho Chi MInh City from the Bitexco Financial tower

Further north of the Mekong Delta live multiple pockets of Cham, Khmer and other ethnic minority communities. This region is also home to many Viet followers of religious sects such as Hoa Hao Buddhism and Caodaism, which have both been linked to military disputes with ruling powers throughout the twentieth century.[129]

Southern Vietnam has an extreme climate with scorching heat, torrential rains and storms, while the flood plains, mountains and dense wildlife-rich forests make for a hostile environment. These factors coupled with hundreds of years of conflict have ensured a solid tradition of combat systems referred to as "the martial arts of forests and gardens."[130]

To the observer, influences from the Chinese, Khmer, Cham and Viet populations are all visible within the Southern Vietnamese martial arts. Such aspects may be seen within the techniques themselves, the weapons trained, the methods of transmission, the associated religious/spiritual practices or all of the above.

In this chapter we will examine some of the largest martial arts schools and culturally relevant styles developed in this region.

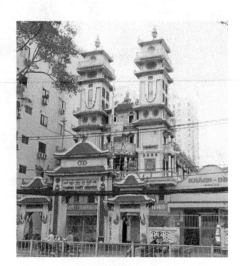

A Cao Dai Temple
in District One, Ho Chi Minh City

BA TRA TAN KHANH / TAKHADO

Võ Lâm Bà Trà Tân Khánh

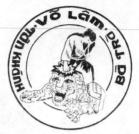

Ba Tra Tan Khanh or Takhado is a martial art that was developed in Binh Duong, a province immediately north of Ho Chi Minh City. The name *Bà Trà* refers to a local hero and skilled fighter, **Lady Tra** of *Tân Khánh* Village, while *Takhado* means (*Tan Khanh Style*).

The school's logo is based on the story of two brothers and teachers of the style named Vo Van At and Vo Van Gia. According to local legend, the pair became famous for defeating live tigers in the relatively-common attacks that happened on villages throughout the pre-industrialized Mekong Delta.[131]

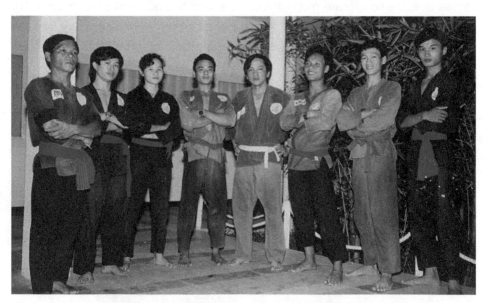

Fig. 21. A young Master Ho Tuong with his students of Ba Tra Tan Khanh

HISTORY

According to Master Ho Tuong, during the early seventeenth century, a number of Binh Dinh Province inhabitants were forced from their homelands by monarchical oppression and a lack of natural resources, such as wood to build houses and animals to hunt. These pioneers ventured south where they established a new village and named it Tan Khanh—now known as Tan Phuoc Khanh Town, Tan Uyen District, Binh Duong Province.

The new citizens of Binh Duong Province had to adjust to their environment and are said to have utilized their martial arts skills to face new and dangerous enemies, including wild predators, marauding bands of thieves and an unforgiving landscape. In many cases this meant disregarding old techniques and creating or adapting new ones that were better suited to their altered needs and environment.[132]

In Tan Khanh Village, a local tea stall owner, martial arts expert and alleged descendant of the Tay Son Rebels named Vo Thi Tra, led an uprising against the ruling authorities of the region. The rebellion managed to hold off their oppressors from regaining control for more than nine years before succumbing to the recently arrived, more powerful and well-equipped French colonial rulers in 1859.[133]

While the inciting incidents for the rebellion are unclear and different sources provide different accounts, possible explanations may have been in response to governmental corruption, high taxes or even as a result of disputes between local ethnic groups such as the Khmer and the relatively new Viet settlers to the region. What is known however, is that during this time the martial arts style of the region adopted its name from Lady (Ba) Tra's Tan Khanh Rebellion.[134]

As time went on, numerous famous martial artists emerged from the region, solidifying the village's reputation as a hotspot of martial prowess. In particular, Master Bay Phien who trained students for the anti-French resistance movement and (future Grandmaster) Ho Van Lanh, a highly regarded Ba Tra Tan Khanh martial artist, who moved from Binh Duong Province to Saigon and became instrumental in the expansion of the style throughout Vietnam and abroad. [135]

Currently, Ba Tra Tan Khanh style is taught all over Vietnam. The largest followings are in Ho Chi Minh City (with over one hundred masters), as well as the southern provinces of Binh Duong, Dong Nai, Dong Thap and Kien Giang.

Although based primarily in Vietnam, due to the dispersion of many southern citizens following the Second Indochina War, a number of Ba Tra Tan Khanh students have continued to teach in the United States, Australia, France and other European countries.

The main representative of Ba Tra Tan Khanh in Vietnam is Master Ho Tuong, the youngest son of Grandmaster Ho Van Lanh. The school's headquarters are based at the Youth Culture House, Pham Ngoc Thach Street, Ben Nghe Ward, District One, Ho Chi Minh City.

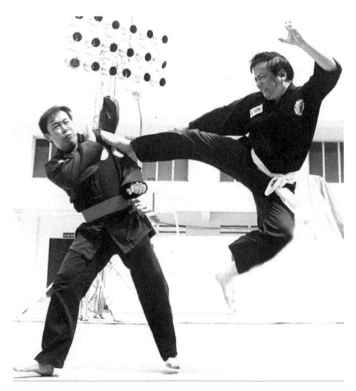

Fig. 22. Master Ho Tuong demonstrates a flying kick

CHARACTERISTICS

Master Ho Tuong describes the syllabus of Ba Tra Tan Khanh martial arts to include: basic strength and conditioning exercises, forms, pair drills which focus on automating reactions and kinesthetic awareness, *Qigong*, competitive fighting and weapons training.[136]

As the Ba Tra Tan Khanh style has its roots in Binh Dinh region martial arts, there are a number of similarities that can be observed. These include: low and high angles of attack that combine deep grounded stances and aerial strikes; frequent leg kicks and stamps; as well as circular and evasive footwork that focuses on avoiding enemy strikes and redirecting momentum—similar to those found in Tai Chi or Aikido.

In comparison to Vo Co Truyen and the Binh Dinh region martial arts, Master Ho identifies the unique aspects of the Ba Tra Tan Khanh style to include:

- "A prioritized focus on pairwork—forms are often trained with live opponents rather than individually to ensure self-defense skills are kept sharp.

- Weapon training with short sticks as well as longer staffs. They are primarily utilized to counterattack by controlling the space and direction of the conflict rather than staying out of range.

- Several empty-handed forms that emphasize quick forward and backward motions, rather than circular movements; these add variety to the fighter's arsenal.

- Stances that focus on constant transition between movements, rather than holding positions for aesthetic purposes.

- A set of thirty-two basic weapons, including various farming and everyday implements that have been absorbed into the style through necessity.

- Forms that are taught through heavily-coded sets of poetry and rhymes—although this method of tuition is used in various Vo Co Truyen schools, it is especially emphasized in the Ba Tra Tan Khanh style (the regional accent and vocabulary also lend themselves well to this purpose).

- A focus on studying the theory of attacks and forms before learning the physical movements (this contrasts many martial arts styles in which the movements are taught first and then analyzed later on)."[137]

Ba Tra Tan Khanh students wear similar attire to that of other Vo Co Truyen schools. Predominantly black, long-sleeved shirts and pants, with a sash of either blue, red, yellow or white indicating their levels as beginner, student, teacher or master respectively. The school's logo is always on the front of the shirts and is often accompanied by the name of the student and specific training location, which makes practitioners of this style easily recognizable.

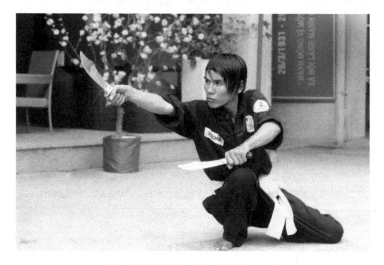

Fig. 23. Ba Tra Tan Khanh knife attack

Benefits of Ba Tra Tan Khanh training

- Flexible Weaponry: The style emphasizes training with unconventional weapons. This may be beneficial in self-defense scenarios.

- Accessibility in Vietnam: As one of the largest single-style martial arts organizations in the South of the country, it is easy to find places to train, particularly in and around Ho Chi Minh City.

- Quality of training: As the head of the organization, Master Ho Tuong oversees many of the Ba Tra Tan Khanh clubs personally, ensuring they are consistent and well managed. Master Ho is truly passionate about martial arts and incredibly welcoming to all visitors, Vietnamese or foreign.

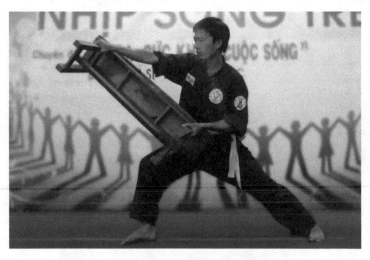

Fig. 24. A student demonstrates one of the everyday implements included in training

SA LONG CUONG
MARTIAL ARTS SCHOOL

Võ Phái Bình Định Sa Long Cương

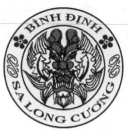

Fig. 25.

Sa Long Cuong is an offshoot of Binh Dinh region martial arts that was popularized in the south of the country. The style is thought to have begun as a blended system of various Vietnamese and Chinese martial arts, which were then adapted for the local population by Grandmaster Truong Thanh Dang in the early twentieth century.[138]

The name *Sa Long Cương* is often translated as *Dragon in the Sand* and refers to the School's founder, who hails from the coastal region of Phan Thiet, Binh Thuan Province.

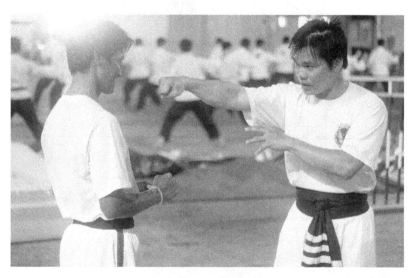

*Master Nguyen Thanh Bao
demonstrates punching techniques during a class in Ho Chi Minh City*

History

The style begins with Truong Thanh Dang who was born into a family with a strong martial arts background in 1894. At the age of fourteen, he was sent by his parents to formally study martial arts in Binh Dinh Province.

After arriving in Binh Dinh, Truong Thanh Dang is said to have trained with several masters, including a Shaolin specialist named Vinh Phuc and most notably, Truong Thach, a descendant of the Truong Clan who first documented the region's martial arts.[139] At the time, the French colonial government had a strict prohibition on martial arts so all training had to be carried out surreptitiously and through informal mentoring.

Truong Thanh Dang spent years researching and honing the techniques he had learned from the various great masters of Vietnamese styles. Then, from 1925–1930, he began to consolidate the techniques he had studied into an orthodox system. Due to the continued prohibition of martial arts, Truong Thanh Dang had to move from the coastal Phan Thiet Province, where he had been teaching for the last five years, to Saigon (Ho Chi Minh City) in 1930, where he was relatively unknown and could teach without drawing unwanted attention.

Dang continued to teach informally up until 1964 when he officially formed the Binh Dinh-Sa Long Cuong school. The organization expanded with great success up until Grandmaster Truong's death in 1985, at the age of ninety-one. His oldest son Truong Ba Duong and the school's director Le Van Van continued to teach and promote the style, maintaining the traditions and history of Truong Thanh Dang's legacy.[140]

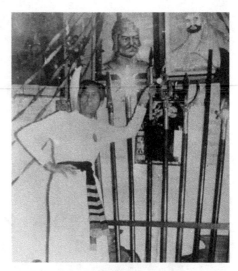

Fig. 26. Grandmaster Truong Thanh Dang alongside pictures of Quang Trung and Bodhidharma

Sa Long Cuong is one of the largest single-style organizations of Vietnamese traditional martial arts, with thousands of practitioners throughout Vietnam, France, Italy, Russia, Canada and the Americas.[141] They are official representatives of the Vo Co Truyen Association of Vietnam and often host foreign and domestic contests and exchanges throughout the country.

CHARACTERISTICS

Master Nguyen Thanh Bao describes the typical progression of Sa Long Cuong students as first learning punching, kicking and **Qigong** routines to work on their balance, strength, and flexibility. Following this, they focus on unarmed forms and self-defense applications that combine the above into combat practice, before moving onto weapons training.[142]

Despite sharing some forms with Vo Co Truyen schools such as: *Lão Mai Quyền* (*Plum Blossom Form*) and *Lão Hổ Thượng Sơn* (*Wise Tiger Ascending The Mountain*), many of those taught in the Sa Long Cuong style appear more linear and less embellished than their Binh Dinh counterparts—the intention of the founder may have been to simplify form training with a view to enable students to learn quickly and effectively.

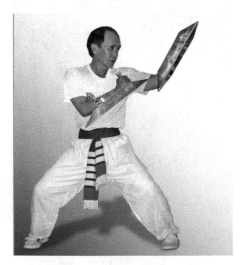
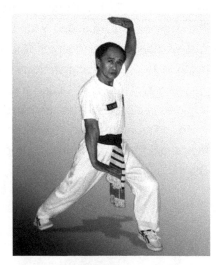

Fig. 27-28. Master Le Van Van demonstrates Song Xi and open-handed techniques

While many fundamentals of the two systems are similar, according to Master Nguyen there are several key differences. The Sa Long Cuong style downplays the use of jumping techniques and prefers to stay grounded, whereas many Binh Dinh styles heavily emphasize aerial attacks. The Sa Long Cuong style also stresses the importance of keeping the arms in a tight guard—closer to the body—this offers more protection and highlights an important principle of never overextending during attacks.[143]

Sa Long Cuong students train with a wide variety of weapons—including the traditional eighteen of Vo Co Truyen and others. The practice of **Song Xi** (**Double Blades**) is common as both a defensive and offensive tool and Sa Long Cuong practitioners also train with long staffs—around three meters. This method of long-staff fighting utilizes the weapon primarily as a linear stabbing and striking implement as opposed to a more circular defensive tool. This draws parallels to other systems (such as Wing Chun) that feature weapons of a similar length.[144] Master Nguyen considers that this particular size staff within Sa Long Cuong was originally used for fending off mounted attackers by serving as a tool for stabbing at the horse.

Sa Long Cuong uniforms are usually white; this comes from the attire of the Nguyen Dynasty generals—they would often wear white when at home, which eventually came to represent their outfits for training. Belts come in four colors: black, blue, red and yellow. The yellow belt shows various degrees of mastery which are represented with up to nine red stripes across the belt before reaching full-yellow.[145]

BENEFITS OF SA LONG CUONG TRAINING

- Accessibility outside of Vietnam: There are schools of Sa Long Cuong in several European countries and the organization is extremely active in the development of international tournaments, exchanges and events.

- Training methodology: The Sa Long Cuong style emphasizes traditional, yet functional training. For example, forms are often taught in a manner that focuses on practical application rather than performance characteristics, while sparring is done with minimal protection to ensure realism.

NAM HUYNH DAO
MARTIAL ARTS SCHOOL

Môn Phái Nam Huỳnh Đạo

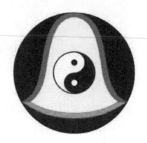

Fig. 29.

The Nam Huynh Dao Martial Arts School is based in District One, Ho Chi Minh City. The name refers to the *Huynh Family Lineage* of martial arts while *Đạo* means the *way* or *path*.

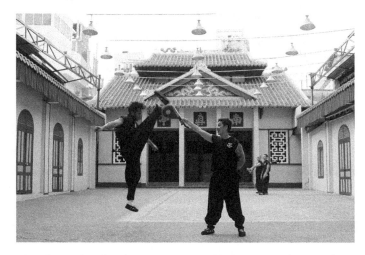

An advanced student demonstrating aerial kicks at Nam Chon Temple in Ho Chi Minh City

HISTORY

According to the association of Nam Huynh Dao, the family martial arts lineage was founded by General Nguyen Huynh Duc, a former viceroy to the southern states of the nation under the Nguyen Dynasty (1748–1819). Huynh Duc was known far and wide for both his martial arts and military skills; in 1997 his mausoleum in Long An Province (southwest of Ho Chi Minh City) was designated as an official historical monument.[146]

The current Grandmaster, named Huynh Tuan Kiet, is the seventh-generation descendant of General Nguyen Huynh Duc. He was taught the family style of martial arts through a paternal lineage, as well as traditional medicines and philosophy by his grandfather (who was a well-known physician of Long An Province).[147]

In a bid to develop the style further, Kiet is said to have combined his family's martial arts with training elements of popular Chinese martial arts such as Choy Li Fut and Choy Gar. With this combination of combatives and traditional medicines, Kiet's family lineage expanded into a comprehensive system and formed the modern style of Nam Huynh Dao. The school officially opened on September 16th, 1991 in their first location at the Nam Chon Temple in District One, Ho Chi Minh City.[148]

In recent years, the Nam Huynh Dao school has been the center of some controversy surrounding online videos of Grandmaster Huynh Tuan Kiet performing seemingly impossible feats (such as no-touch knockouts) using only *Qi*, as well as the schools' cult-like appearance.[149] Despite attracting a large amount of backlash from the online martial arts community for such practices, during the author's own experiences visiting training sessions and researching the style in-person, the practices observed were typical martial arts techniques and traditional training methodologies, all taught and demonstrated by skilled instructors and disciples.

CHARACTERISTICS

Training sessions in the school headquarters at Nam Chon Temple focus heavily on physical conditioning. They include routines of strengthening stances, working on flexibility and developing explosive striking power through combinations of techniques performed in lines moving through the courtyard. Open-handed strikes, punches, throws and sweeps make up the core sets of techniques used within practice.

Alongside martial techniques, softer elements of breath control, meditation and *Qigong* are also present within the Nam Huynh Dao syllabus; sessions that focus on these aspects attract many older practitioners wishing to develop health and fitness.

Philosophy and the study of traditional medicines are also considered to be cornerstones of the Nam Huynh Dao School and are highly emphasized as part of its pedagogy.[150]

During formal training sessions, students dress in black pants and sleeveless black shirts or t-shirts. They wear yellow, red, blue or white colored sashes denoting ranks as low-level students, high-level students, instructors or masters. Practitioners wear light, material footwear similar to those often worn by monks and many senior students also shave their heads, adding further to their monk-like appearance.

Benefits of Nam Huynh Dao training

- Fitness: Training sessions are extremely intense and fitness focused. They practice a whole range of cardiovascular conditioning, flexibility, endurance and strength training in every session.

- Mental training: The Nam Huynh Dao style strongly emphasizes the non-physical aspects of training, particularly developing focus, determination and dedication among students (training sessions begin at four o'clock each morning).

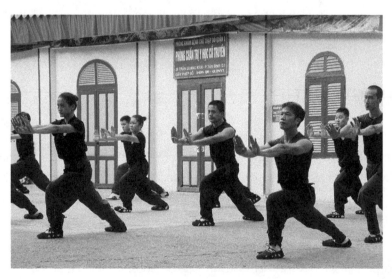

Students practice palm-striking techniques

SEVEN MOUNTAINS MARTIAL ARTS

Võ Miền Bảy Núi

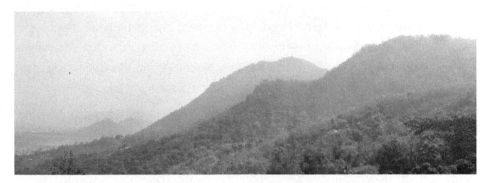

The view of Forbidden Mountain—the largest of the range

Võ Miền translates as *Martial Arts* while *Bảy Núi* literally means *Seven Mountains* (a range that lies close to the Cambodian border in An Giang Province—about two hundred and fifty kilometers west of Ho Chi Minh City). The name refers to various lineages of martial arts practiced by Buddhist and Daoist groups in the region.

The terrain of Seven Mountains includes a mix of densely forested peaks and low-lying floodplains that are annually overrun with water from the Mekong River and its many tributaries. As a result, boats are often the preferred method of everyday transport among the floating markets and villages built on stilts over waterways.

Due to the treacherous landscape and variety of dangerous animals, such as snakes, tigers, centipedes, bears and crocodiles, the region has historically been extremely isolated. Until the arrival of modern infrastructure and development projects orchestrated by the French and later Vietnamese regimes, the Seven Mountains region was virtually inaccessible to vehicles; often seen as a frontier-land, a place of secrecy and mystery, in particular the highest of the peaks, *Núi Cấm* (*Forbidden Mountain*).[151]

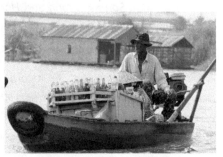

A floating café in An Giang Province Southwest Vietnam

History

Due to a combination of the Seven Mountains' location and history, the population of the area is composed of a diverse mix of ethnic Vietnamese, Hoa, Cham and Khmer. Although the Seven Mountains were a part of the Khmer Kingdom for hundreds of years, by the early-eighteenth century the first ethnically Vietnamese immigrants began to settle in the region. With them, it is likely that they brought their own martial traditions, which over time mixed with those of the population who "the Vietnamese regarded as strange and bizarre forest peoples." [152]

During pre-colonial times, the culture of the Seven Mountains region was heavily influenced by spiritual practices—somewhat similar to Japanese Shinto—in which spirits manifest themselves in places, objects and creatures. Here, it was not uncommon (and is still not) for communities to incorporate possession ceremonies, spiritual healers and wandering monks into such religious practices. Although this is not entirely unique to the Seven Mountains region, frequent threats from war, dangerous animals and an incredibly hostile environment, combined with a long-lasting tradition of deity and spirit veneration, meant many of the local martial arts practices were developed with both physical combat training and spiritual training in mind. As Tran states, the Seven Mountains martial arts style "evolved not only in response to the human battlefield, but also to combat the invisible powers of the unknown and supernatural." [153]

Throughout the twentieth century, the turbulent political climate resulting from the efforts of factious parties to consolidate their power, (such as the French colonial government, the Catholic regime of President Ngo Dinh Diem and the Communist party), led to the persecution of many religious and ethnic groups of the Seven Mountains region. This, in turn, contributed to the growth of various millenarian Buddhist groups such as the *Bửu Sơn Kỳ Hương* and *Hòa Hảo* Sects—both of which were inspired by the teachings of Doan Minh Huyen or *Phật Thầy* (*Buddha Master*), who was known as a wandering Buddhist healer, holy man and martial arts adept. [154]

Although there are no detailed records of Doan Minh Huyen performing martial arts, many of his disciples were known as skilled warriors. Of these disciples, several later took up arms against the French imperialists (among various other battles and insurrections) and are identified as masters of the Seven Mountains style of martial arts.

One of the best known was Master Tran Van Thanh, a self-appointed successor of the **Buddha Master**. Thanh is considered to have been both a formidable practitioner of Khmer martial arts and Shamanism, as well as a Commander of the Nguyen Dynasty military before joining Doan Minh Huyen's congregation.[155]

After the death of his teacher, Tran Van Thanh is said to have led a force of twelve hundred combined Khmer and Viet frontiersmen in an uprising against the Colonial French powers equipped with only hand weapons and their martial arts skills. "The Army of the Mountains," as they were known, held off the French from 1867-1873, before finally being overpowered by the might of modern artillery. Thanh's army was quickly disbanded and some sources state that their leader was killed in battle, while others suggest that he simply disappeared into the wilderness.[156]

In more recent years, many of the spiritual and martial arts practices of the region were prohibited or threatened by conflict but remained taught in the isolation of the mountains.[157] Even to this day, the attributes of the Seven Mountains' geomancy or **Phong Thuỷ** (**Feng Shui**) are believed by inhabitants to instill in them a heightened sense of spiritual vitality and the region is still seen by many as a mysterious holy land.[158]

There are various groups of Buddhists and Daoists still in the region and across Vietnam that practice the Seven Mountains martial arts. Due to the dispersion of the population following periods of war and oppression, there are also similar traditions among Khmer and Vietnamese groups in the United States and European countries.

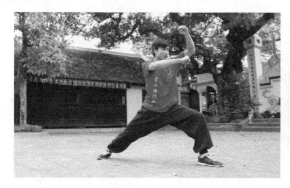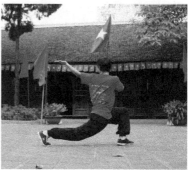

A "Mountain" and "Snake" stance of Seven Mountains region martial arts

CHARACTERISTICS

The Seven Mountains martial arts styles are typically centered around forms based upon the movements of animals and/or powerful spirits. These include numerous types such as the Tiger, Crane, Hawk, Snake, Monkey, Phoenix and Dragon.[159]

In the author's own experiences of Seven Mountains martial arts, a number of techniques are reminiscent of typical Southeast Asian and Khmer styles. These include a focus on the close-range use of elbows, knees and headbutts, while other aspects are more frequently seen in Northern Vietnamese and Chinese styles such as wide and low stances and high, long-range kicks. Similarly, weapons practiced in these systems vary widely but often incorporate both Chinese-style battlefield tools—such as swords, spears and axes—and those more typical of Southeast Asian fighting systems such as daggers, short sticks and concealed blades similar to the *Karambit*.[160]

Furthermore, techniques in the Seven Mountains style are generally taught with realism in mind; in particular, there are few sporting or competitive adaptations that might detract from the fundamentally practical nature of the style.

Many forms of the Seven Mountains martial arts share similarities with Chinese styles in that they draw inspiration from animals. However, a key difference is that practitioners of the Seven Mountains martial arts do not try to learn physical techniques based on imitating the movements of the animals, but rather attempt to embody the "spirit" of the creature and allow it to animate their movements.[161]

The Seven Mountains martial arts forms can be performed as set routines of functional, combative techniques (in the same vein as those utilized by Shaolin or Vo Co Truyen practitioners), however, adept practitioners may improvise forms. This can be likened this to a dancer who "does not premeditate a sequence of movements."[162] Forms may also be practiced in veneration of particular spirits or deities—something which might appear to outside observers as a form of spirit possession (a belief not uncommon in some strands of Vietnamese folk-religion).

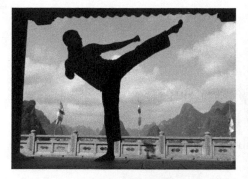 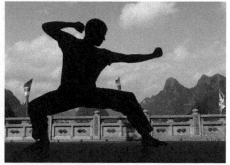

A practitioner of Seven Mountains martial arts demonstrates the dynamic nature of the style

Although the Seven Mountains martial arts are well known in southern Vietnam, it should be noted that these systems, for the most part, have not gone through the same process of modernization as other styles have.

There is no governing body or official ranking system, other than those developed by individual schools or the titles designated from the Buddhist or Daoist clergy upon their disciples.

As these styles are known for their spiritual and cultural importance alongside their physical practices, many Buddhist and Daoist practitioners tend to wear robes or the simple cotton attire of initiated laymen as they train, while other groups may train shirtless to beat the sweltering heat of the region or simply in their everyday attire.

BENEFITS OF SEVEN MOUNTAINS STYLE TRAINING

- Spirituality: The region itself (and related martial practices) are closely connected with both Buddhist and Daoist practices. Many schools of Seven Mountains martial arts incorporate both physical and spiritual practices such as meditation, *Qigong* and philosophy.

- Traditional methodology: Due to the roots of the style, training monks and warriors in the dense wilderness and extreme climate of south Vietnam, training in the Seven Mountains martial arts can often be extremely intense and physically challenging.

KHMER MARTIAL ARTS

Võ Thuật Khmer

The Khmer are known for their long history as warriors, much of their combat legacy is detailed within the carvings in ancient Cambodian temples such as **Angkor Wat** and the walled city of **Angkor Thom**.[163]

For centuries the Khmer dominated large parts of Southeast Asia, however, in modern-day Vietnam they make up less than one percent of the population and as a result, the forms of martial arts practiced by the Vietnamese Khmer (Khmer Krom) are limited in comparison to those of neighboring Cambodia. However, certain groups are working to ensure the Khmer Krom martial arts culture remains strong.

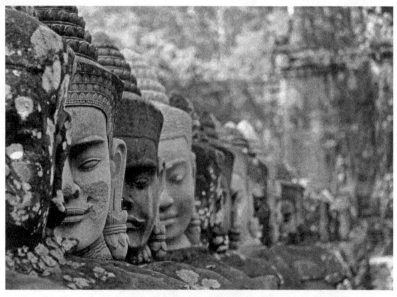

The Khmer warrior guards outside the gates of Angkor Thom

HISTORY

From the tenth to eighteenth centuries the Vietnamese empire was continually and aggressively expanding southwards. Over hundreds of years and through numerous wars with the Khmer Empire (who were at their height of power between 802–1431 CE), the Viet managed to gradually assume control of the southern provinces.

While many of the Khmer population based around the Mekong Delta receded into Cambodia over time, a small number remained, currently there are around a million. Over the years, the Khmer Krom were involved in numerous uprisings and conflicts with the Viet, French, Siamese and other oppositions. Tales and legends of Khmer martial artists in the region are widespread, such as that of Pu Kombo, a claimant to the throne of the Khmer Kingdom who led the Khmer forces in Tran Van Thanh's uprising. Another is the Buddhist Master Ta Paul who was allegedly tortured, poisoned and boiled alive at the hands of the French but appeared unkillable.[164] The latter draws parallels to other folk heroes across the globe, such as Rasputin who was allegedly both stabbed and poisoned seemingly without effect.

Throughout the twentieth century, the region was in constant turmoil, and eventually culminated with a Viet invasion of Cambodia against the Khmer Rouge—prolific for their orchestration of the Cambodian genocide from 1975–1979. In more recent years, the Khmer Krom remain the subject of Human Rights debates, particularly in regards to the way that they have been forced to adopt Vietnamese names, language and customs in an attempt to better assimilate into Vietnamese culture and social systems.[165] This cultural prohibition may be largely responsible for the lack of widespread Khmer Krom martial arts practices in Vietnam today, however some small schools remain.

In Tra Cu Village (known in Khmer as **Preah Trapeng**), Tra Vinh Province, a master known by the Vietnamese name of Thach Thanh teaches his family's traditional martial arts style. According to Thach, he was trained by his grandfather, a famous martial artist and activist in the region named My Son.[166]

Currently, Master Thach Thanh's school has dozens of local students; to whom he also teaches Khmer language and traditional dance. He is extremely active in promoting the culture of the Khmer Krom martial arts and his students can often be seen in cultural exhibitions and displays throughout the southern provinces.

For the time being at least, Master Thanh's school and others like it ensure the preservation of practices from a once dominant culture in Vietnam, that are now verging on extinction.

CHARACTERISTICS

Although the Khmer Empire was heavily influenced by Indian cultural and religious practices, it has been suggested that the martial arts "statues and relief figures portrayed more closely resemble Chinese boxing stances than any known arts of India."[167] It is thought that the reasons for this may be attributed to the common heritage of modern-day Cambodia with countries such as Thailand and Vietnam, that have been more heavily influenced by Chinese culture.

Regardless of historical influences, Khmer martial arts are still practiced in southern Vietnam and Cambodia as methods of self-defense, performance pieces and as a tool for religious and spiritual cultivation.

To the observer, the modern martial arts of the Khmer Krom appear almost identical to the Cambodian system of **Bokator** (which translates as **Pounding the Lion**) and was developed as an amalgamated style of Khmer martial arts early in the twenty-first century. This system incorporates aspects of "pradal serey" kickboxing, traditional wrestling and animal-style forms, as well as weapons."[168]

From the author's own experiences, the unarmed styles of Khmer Krom martial arts heavily emphasize close-range striking; using the hands, feet, elbows knees and even headbutts, as well as joint locking and immobilization techniques. In these respects, the Khmer Krom systems share common ground with other types of Southeast Asian combatives such as **Muay Boran** (Traditional Thai Boxing) or **Bando** (Burmese Boxing). However, regional variations have likely adapted between the groups of practitioners in Vietnam and Cambodia, who in a border-free reimagining of the region would essentially be different clans of the same people.

The practice attire of the Khmer Krom martial arts is simple, usually consisting of just shorts and hand-wraps (typically wound rope), with a **Krama** (**Scarf**) tied around the head as a bandanna and around the waist.

BENEFITS OF KHMER MARTIAL ARTS

- Effectiveness—For the Khmer Krom, much like their Cambodian counterparts, there is little room for frivolity and the practice of forms and aesthetically pleasing moves are often downplayed while effective knockout or severe-injury strikes are emphasized.

- Range—While the Khmer Krom martial arts heavily feature close-range striking, they also utilize transition-range techniques (i.e. standing grapples/throws/sweeps) with great effect. This allows practitioners to continue fighting without much emphasis on ground grappling.

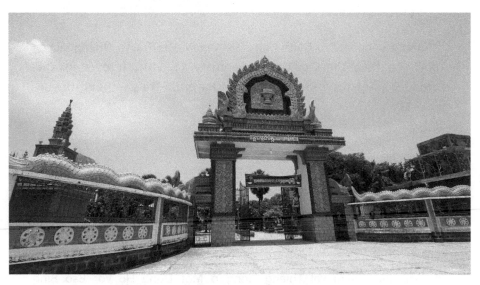

A Khmer temple in An Giang province, Southwest Vietnam

CHAPTER FOUR NOTES

[128] Lam, Fai Chun, "Preamble on the Origin and Development of Hung Kuen." *Journal of Chinese Martial Studies*, no. 1 (January 1, 2009), 55.

[129] Taylor, K W., *A History of the Vietnamese*, (Cambridge: Cambridge University Press, 2013), 537.

[130] Ngoc Huu and Lady Borton, *Martial Arts—Võ Dân Tộc*, (Hanoi, Thế Giới Publishers, 2005), 35.

[131] Ibid., 57.

[132] Ho Tuong, Master Ba Tra Tan Khanh School, in discussion with the author, The Youth Cultural House, District One, Ho Chi Minh City, April 2016.

[133] Ibid.

[134] Cuong Phuong, "Võ Đánh Cọp 'Tân Khánh—Bà Trà' Và Những Huyền Thoại," An Ninh The Gioi Online, February 11, 2016, http://antg.cand. com.vn/Phong-su/Vo-danh-cop-Tan-Khanh-Ba-Tra-va-nhung-huyen-thoai-381591/.

[135] Ibid.

[136] Ho, in discussion with the author, 2016.

[137] Ibid.

[138] Nguyen Tuyen Kim, "Bình Định Sa Long Cương Trong Tầm Vóc Mới," Bao Binh Dinh, September 29, 2006, http://www.baobinhdinh.com.vn/Butkyphongsu/ 2006/9/33093/.

[139] Khai Nhan, "Báu Vật Thiêng Liêng ở Một Dòng Họ Võ," Bao Binh Dinh, September 1, 2006, http://www.baobinhdinh.com.vn/Disan-dulich/2006/9/31897/.

[140] Sa Long Cuong France, "School System of Sa Long Cuong Martial Arts," 2014, http://www.binhdinh-salongcuong.org /GB_HISTORY_School System_Vo-Tran Binh-Dinh Tay-Son.html.

[141] Nguyen,"Bình Định Sa Long Cương," 2006.

[142] Nguyen Thanh Bao, Sa Long Cuong School Master, in discussion with the author, The Youth Cultural House, District One, Ho Chi Minh City, April 2016.

[143] Nguyen, in discussion with the author, 2016.

[144] Kwok Wing Chun, "The Martial Art Syllabus," 2020, http://www.kwokwingchun.com/.

[145] Sa Long Cuong France, "Ranks and Degrees," 2014, http://www.binhdinh-salongcuong.org/GB_ MARTIAL%20ARTS_Ranks%20and%20Degrees.html.

[146] Vuong Hong Thu, "Giới Thiệu," Nam Huỳnh Đạo, Accessed January 31, 2020, http://namhuynhdao.vn/gioi-thieu.

[147] Vo Thuat, "Giải Mã Môn Võ Việt Có Thể 'Lấy Một Địch Mười'," August 6, 2015, http://www.vothuat.vn/cac-mon-phai/giai-ma-mon-vo-viet-co-lay-mot-dich-muoi.html.

[148] Vuong, "Giới Thiệu," n.d.

[149] Tien Phong, "Nam Huỳnh Đạo: Môn Võ Bí Hiểm Bậc Nhất Việt Nam," VTC News, June 7, 2017, https://vtc.vn/the-thao/do-nhap-vo-duong-nam-huynh-dao-ar328294.html.

[150] Vo Thuat, "Giải Mã Môn".

[151] Nong Son Huyen, "Huyền Thoại Võ Phái Thất Sơn Thần Quyền," An Ninh The Gioi Online, May 5, 2011, http://antg.cand.com.vn/Phong-su/Hu"yen-thoai-vo-phai- That-Son-Than-Quyen-300215/.

[152] Tran, Jason Hoai, "Than Quyen: An Introduction to Spirit Forms of That Son Vietnamese Martial Arts." *Journal of Asian Martial Arts* 13, no. 2 (2004): 65–78. 67.

[153] Ibid., 67.

[154] Thich, Quang Huyen, *Dharma Mountain Buddhism & Martial Yoga*, (Frederick, MD: Dharma Mountain Publications, Chùa Xá Lợi 2010).

[155] Ibid., 88-95.

[156] Ibid.

[157] Nong, "Huyền Thoại Võ".

[158] Tran, "Than Quyen".

[159] Ibid.

[160] The Karambit is a short curved dagger found throughout Malay, Indonesian and Filipino martial arts.

[161] Thich, *Dharma Mountain*, 353-362.

[162] Ibid., 358.

[163] Green, Thomas A., *Martial Arts of the World: An Encyclopedia*, (Santa Barbara, CA: ABC-CLIO, 2001), 541.

[164] Thich, *Dharma Mountain*, 115.

[165] Adams, Brad, Bill Frelick, Dinah Po Kempner, and Joseph Saunders, *On the Margins: Rights Abuses of Ethnic Khmer in Vietnam's Mekong Delta*, (New York: Human Rights Watch, 2009).

[166] Khanh Phuong, "Võ Khmer Phục Hồi ở Trà Vinh," Tien Phong, April 3, 2006, https://www.tienphong.vn/the-thao /vo-khmer-phuc-hoi-o-tra-vinh-39900.tpo.

[167] Green, *Martial Arts of the World*, 541.

[168] Antionio Graceffo, "The Battle to Preserve Cambodia's Martial Arts Heritage," Black Belt, July 1, 2019, https://blackbeltmag.com/arts/history-philosophy/bokator-forever, para. 6.

CHAPTER FOUR FIGURES

Chapter V

FOREIGN MARTIAL ARTS IN VIETNAM

As we have seen, the martial arts systems that have arisen within the borders of Vietnam cannot be easily attributed to any sole culture or ethnicity. Instead, they can be considered as being derived from a wide variety of peoples and influences.

Historically, China in particular, has had a profound effect upon the development of Vietnamese martial arts. This influence remains to the present day, with numerous modern (post-nineteenth century) Chinese martial arts systems still practiced widely in Vietnam.

Similarly, other nations that have once held a presence in Vietnam continue to exert their influence on modern-day martial arts practices, such as Japan, Korea and even Western nations.

In recent years, foreign martial arts have come to represent an important part of modern Vietnamese culture, particularly among the younger generation. Many see foreign martial arts as a tool to bridge perceived divides between the Vietnamese people and the rest of the world or as progressive ways for local citizens to embody the warrior ideals that have become part of the Vietnamese national identity.

In this chapter, we will consider the most significant and widely followed foreign martial arts systems practiced in Vietnam.

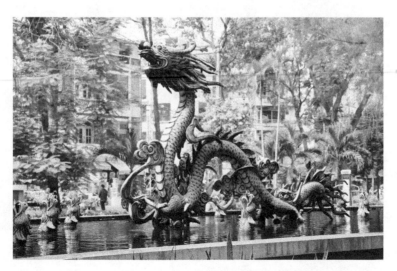

A dragon monument marking the center of Saigon's Chinatown

HUNG GAR KUEN

Hồng Gia Quyền

Hung Gar Kuen is a Southern Chinese martial art style. It is said to be one of five major family schools that were derived directly from Shaolin martial art teachings (others include Choy Gar, Lau Gar, Li Gar and Mok Gar). Hung Gar Kuen became extremely popular throughout China during the late nineteenth and early twentieth century for a number of reasons, however its association with the widely-known Chinese folk hero Wong Fei Hung is thought to have had a large contribution to this.[168]

Some of the earliest noted observations of **Hồng Gia Quyền** (as it is known in Vietnam), were during the early twentieth century in the Cholon (Chinatown) District of Ho Chi Minh City. Several schools from this area trace the emergence of the style back to a Chinese Master named Huynh Thuan Quy, who worked as a leather tanner in the Cholon market.[169]

Currently, Hong Gia Quyen has a large following around both the Red River Delta and the Mekong Delta, with hundreds of schools and many thousands of students. One Ho Chi Minh City-based school claims to have trained over five hundred instructors alone.[170]

The practical nature and adaptability of Hong Gia Quyen, along with the physicality of the training, are likely to have assisted with its spread throughout Vietnam; self-defense skills and physical fitness are key benefits for those at risk during periods of conflict.

Many practices commonly associated with Hong Gia Quyen training have since been incorporated into various traditional Vietnamese martial art schools, some examples of which are strengthening the fingers by striking a bucket of sand or gravel, or training drills with iron rings worn on the wrists to assist with both forearm conditioning and strengthening of the muscles.[171]

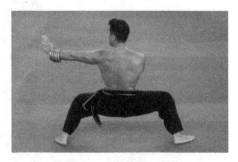

A Hong Gia Quyen practitioner demonstrating iron ring techniques

WING CHUN

Vịnh Xuân Quyền

Due to its accessibility and relative ease of learning, Wing Chun or **Vịnh Xuân Quyền** as the Vietnamese schools are referred to, is extremely popular throughout Vietnam. Thousands of Vinh Xuan schools from various lineages are distributed across the country.

Although Wing Chun famously originated in southern China and was popularized in Hong Kong during the 1950s, it is considered to have first developed a significant following in Vietnam near the beginning of the twentieth century. A Chinese master and seventh-generation disciple of the southern Shaolin temple, named Nguyen Te Cong, is credited with its introduction into the nation.[172] Despite the likelihood that alternative lineages of Vinh Xuan may have been taught in Vietnamese-Chinese communities before this, Nguyen Te Cong was the first to bring the system to mainstream recognition in Vietnam.

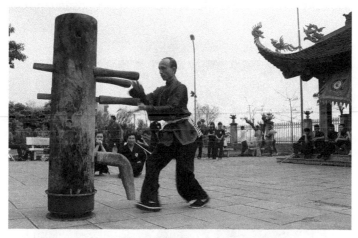

A Vinh Xuan master performing a wooden dummy form

As the school lineages diverged through students of Nguyen Te Cong, the Vietnamese style of Vinh Xuan was further adapted to suit the location and the physicality of its practitioners.[173] From the author's own experiences of Vietnamese Vinh Xuan Quyen some of the key features of style include the following:

- Chain punching (using vertically aligned fists to repeatedly strike forward using the hands alternately in a quick circular motion), sunken elbow defense and upright stances with low kicks. All of these techniques are similar in practice to Hong Kong lineages.

- Heavy arm and leg conditioning. This is often done in a manner similar to that of "external" martial arts, "relying mostly on building up muscle and bone strength."[174]

- Liberal use of high kicks. These are commonly downplayed in Southern-Chinese systems that prefer hand strikes and close-range techniques.

- Clearly represented animal forms. These are absent from the Yip Man/Hong Kong lineage of Wing Chun, which typically features just three unarmed forms.[175]

- Reduced emphasis on the use of wooden dummy practice. This is due in part to the expense and impracticality of the wooden dummy. While a variety of unconventional (and occasionally aggressive) forms of Chi Sao or Sticking Hands are employed instead.[176]

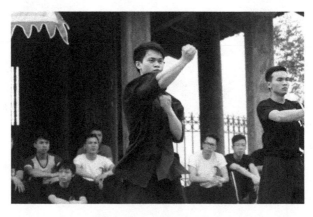

Vinh Xuan Students demonstrate chain punching

Among the thousands of schools of Vinh Xuan Quyen all over Vietnam, specific styles are often named after family titles and are widely advertised with posters and public training sessions in schools, parks and pagodas.

OTHER POPULAR CHINESE ARTS

A large number of other, contemporary Chinese martial arts have been introduced to Vietnam through immigration and societal crossover, many of which retain large followings. The central hub for Chinese martial art systems is Ho Chi Minh City's Cholon District (which has a huge number of schools), alongside other large cities such as Hanoi, Da Nang, Hue and Nha Trang. The following martial art styles are among the most prevalent:

- *Bak Mei Pai (Bạch Mi Phái)*
  White Eyebrow Kung Fu, named after a Daoist monk from the Emei Mountain region who was famous for his long white beard and eyebrows. The style is said to focus on the use of trapping and close-range hand strikes to vital points.[177]

- *Emei Quan Kung Fu (Võ Phái Nga Mi Sơn)*
  A style of Kung Fu developed on Emei Mountain in Sichuan Province, China. Emei Mountain is known for being one of the most sacred Buddhist and Daoist areas of China. The martial arts styles developed in the mountain's monasteries are famous for emphasizing the use of speed and flexible counter attacks.[178]

- *Fut Gar Kuen (Phật Gia Quyền)*
  Phật Gia Quyền or *Buddhist Family Fist* is a relatively modern style of Kung Fu which was developed as a culmination of various southern Shaolin martial arts schools. It is said to focus on circular footwork with "long powerful whipping and swinging strikes, which utilize both momentum and the whole strength of the body."[179]

- *Tai Chi Chuan (Thái Cực Quyền)*
  An "internal" martial arts style. Tai Chi is particularly popular with older practitioners, as it is commonly practiced with slow movements and offers health benefits in mind as opposed to combat. Tai Chi Chuan, or *Thái Cực Quyền*, practices vary widely between schools. Both the contemporary Chinese lineages (Chen, Sun, Wu, Wu Hao Sun) and those that are considered to be more-distinctly Vietnamese variations remain popular in Vietnam.

- **Wushu**

Wushu is a modern Chinese martial art system featuring two variations, *Taolu* and *Sanda* (*Forms* and *Competitive sparring* respectively). Wushu was developed from an amalgamation of various traditional Chinese martial art systems and has millions of practitioners worldwide. It is often put forward as a bid for inclusion within the summer Olympic Games—although so far has remained unsuccessful.[180]

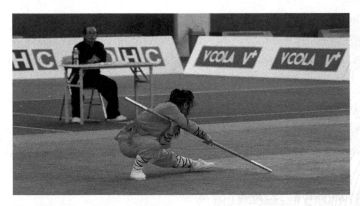

A Vietnamese Shaolin Kung Fu practitioner

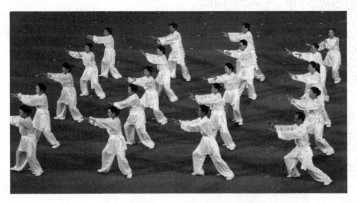

Vietnamese Tai Chi Chuan practitioners

JAPANESE MARTIAL ARTS

Japanese martial arts are immensely popular throughout the world—Judo practitioners alone are estimated to number more than twenty-eight million worldwide.[181] In Vietnam, they are also widespread, with many thousands of practitioners.

Until their surrender in 1945, the Japanese military occupied Vietnam for several years as part of their World War Two conquest of the Pacific. As a result of this occupation, many of the foundations were laid for future cultural and economic trade partnerships. Presently, Japan and Vietnam have a high amount of international trade; Japan has, for several years, been one of the largest investors in Vietnam's manufacturing industry.[182]

Throughout the twentieth century, a significant Japanese population has resided in Vietnam and as a result there are many Vietnamese masters of Japanese martial arts. From the author's own experiences with Japanese martial arts in Vietnam, it is clear that they are especially popular with young people due to the accessibility of the styles as well as the values of respect and discipline that are also important in Vietnamese culture.

Judo has a large following and Vietnamese athletes regularly compete in international contests such as the Southeast Asian Games and Summer Olympics. Some of the most popular Japanese martial arts in Vietnam include:

- **Aikido**
- **Kendo**
- **Goju Ryu Karate**
- **Kyokushin Karate**
- **Judo**
- **Shotokan Karate**

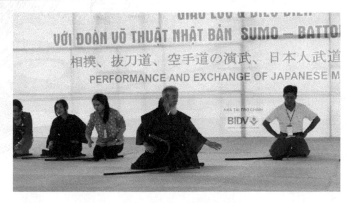

A Japanese sword master demonstrating his art in Vietnam

KOREAN MARTIAL ARTS

Taekwondo is one of the most popular martial arts in the world and is generally divided into two sub-styles:

- **ITF (International Taekwondo Federation)**—Often historically associated with the nation of North Korea.[183]

- **World Taekwondo (WT)** (formerly named **WTF**)—Olympic Style Taekwondo and the national sport of South Korea.

ITF Taekwondo has a large following in Vietnam. Its popularity may be due in part to the cultural exchange between Communist nations, as well as the former Grandmaster Tran Trieu Quan (1952–2010)—a Vietnamese–Canadian from Ho Chi Minh City who served as a high-ranking member of the International Taekwondo Federation from a number of years.[184]

The WT system of Taekwondo is also hugely popular in Vietnam, this may be a result of the numerous South Korean military troops and martial arts instructors stationed in the nation during the Second Indochina War, as well as more recent efforts from South Korea that have sought to develop Taekwondo as an international sport.[185]

Vietnam often hosts Taekwondo events (such as the Asian Open Championships) and submits numerous fighters for events such as the Olympics, South East Asian (SEA) Games and others.

OTHER SOUTHEAST ASIAN MARTIAL ARTS

MUAY THAI

Muay Thai is the national sport of Thailand and is considered by many to be one of the largest Thai cultural exports.[186] Although staging competitive Muay Thai matches in Vietnam has been illegal in the past due to their connections with gambling (which is itself prohibited), in recent years a growing number of professional fights under organizations such as "ONE Championship" have been permitted.

Many Thai citizens and Thai-trained Vietnamese have established gyms and training centers throughout the country and in it is common for practitioners to travel across Southeast Asia to engage in training and competition.

Due to being geographically and culturally accessible to the Vietnamese people, as well as the increasing popularity of Muay Thai in international mixed martial arts events, the sport has accumulated a large and dedicated following in Vietnam.

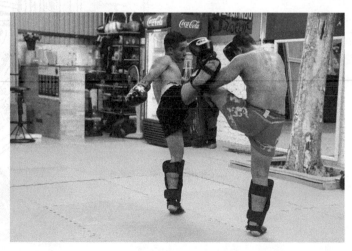

Vietnamese Muay Thai practitioners sparring

PENCAK SILAT

Pencak Silat is an umbrella term for various systems of Indonesian martial arts; this mirrors styles like Vo Co Truyen and Chinese Wushu in which traditional and modern methods have been amalgamated into a uniform, nationalized style.[187]

Pencak Silat has a large following in Vietnam, this may be due to technical and cultural similarities between the Vietnamese and Indonesian martial arts or Pencak Silat's nature as a straight-to-the-point self-defense style as well as an accessible competitive sport.

ESCRIMA/ARNIS

The Filipino stick fighting arts have a significant number of practitioners in Vietnam. The two countries are geographically close, while important trade routes have existed between them for centuries (some scholars even suggest that the Cham may have arrived in Vietnam from the Philippines).[188]

While modern and historic ties between the two nations may account for some level of cultural crossover, the popularity of Escrima and modern Arnis skyrocketed globally after demonstrations of these styles by Bruce Lee and Dan Inosanto in the 1970s. Today there are many Filipino and Vietnamese masters of Escrima/Arnis based throughout the country.

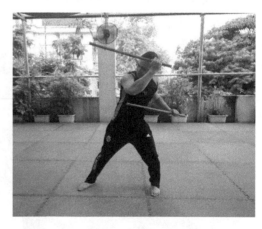

Arnis instructor Gaius Sision teaching a double-stick technique

WESTERN STYLES AND MIXED MARTIAL ARTS

Across Vietnam, much like the rest of the world, the popularity of Mixed Martial Arts (MMA) has grown vastly in recent years. MMA organizations such as the Ultimate Fighting Championship (UFC), ONE Championship, Bellator and others are rapidly becoming some of the most popular televised pay-per-view contests of all time.[189] As a result, the demand for training in MMA is ever-increasing.

In the author's own experience, Boxing, Western Wrestling, Brazilian Jiu Jitsu and Kickboxing are all extremely popular in Vietnam. A growing number of self-defense-oriented styles are also gaining popularity, such as the Israeli Krav Maga and Russian Systema.

Even though these modern styles are developing more of a presence and further saturating an already busy market, they do not necessarily have much impact on the practice of the traditional arts. According to recent research there is a fairly even division between the numbers of traditional and modern martial arts practitioners in Vietnam and each group considers their purposes for training to be different.[190]

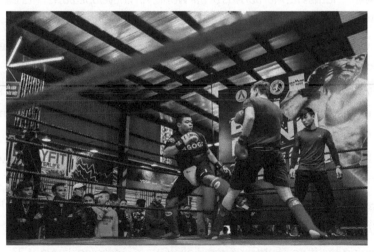

Fig. 30. Competitors in a mixed martial arts event held in Hanoi

CHAPTER FIVE NOTES

[168] Lam, Fai Chun, "Preamble on the Origin and Development of Hung Kuen," *Journal of Chinese Martial Studies*, no. 1 (January 1, 2009), 54.

[169] Thanh Nghia Duong, "Các Môn Phái Thiếu Lâm ở Sài Gòn—Chợ Lớn," 2010, http://thangnghiaduong.com/vo-thuat/cac-mon-phai-thieu-lam-o-sai-gon-cho-lon-9.html.

[170] Anh Vu, "30 Năm 1 Chặng Đường," Hong Gia Quyen VN, August 14, 2011. http://honggiaquyen.vn/page/view/about-us, para. 7.

[171] Taiping Institute, "Hung Kuen," Accessed January 23, 2020, http://taipinginstitute.com/courses/lingnan/hung-kuen.

[172] Ly, "Nguyễn Tế Công—Con Đường Rời Bỏ Trung Hoa Trở Thành Sư Tổ Vịnh Xuân Quyền Việt Nam," Võ Thuật, September 25, 2014, http://www.vothuat.vn/vo-thuat-cuoc-song/nguyen-te-cong-con-duong-roi-bo-trung-hoa-tro-thanh-su-vinh-xuan-quyen-viet-nam.html.

[173] Ibid.

[174] Green, Thomas A., *Martial Arts of the World: An Encyclopedia*, (Santa Barbara, CA: ABC-CLIO, 2001), 38.

[175] Kwok Wing Chun, "The Martial Art Syllabus," 2020, http://www.kwokwingchun.com/.

[176] Sticking hands is a pair-practice exercise in which students strike and block the opponent while maintaining physical contact with each other's forearms, to "sense" where their opponent will strike.

[177] Taiping Institute, "Pak Mei Kuen," Accessed January 23, 2020, http://www.taipinginstitute.com/library/32-uncategorised.

[178] Wang, Guangxi, Chinese Kung Fu, (Cambridge: Cambridge University Press, 2012).

[179] Taiping Institute, "Fut Gar Kuen: Fojia Quan," Accessed January 23, 2020, http://www.taipinginstitute.com/courses/lingnan/fut-gar-kuen, para. 1.

[180] Wang, Chinese Kung Fu, 107.

[181] Tom McGowan and Henry Young, "Inside the World's Most Spiritual Sport," CNN, July 25, 2018, https://edition.cnn.com/2017/12/01/sport/kodokan-institute-noaki-murata-jigoro-kano-tokyo-2020/index.html, para. 26.

[182] Thu Ha, "Japanese Investment in Việt Nam on the Rise in 2019," vietnamnews.vn, April 11, 2019, https://vietnamnews.vn/economy/518583/japanese-investment-in-viet-nam-on-the-rise-in-2019.html.

[183] Dakin R. Burdick, "Korea," in *Martial Arts of the World: An Encyclopedia*, Edited by Thomas A Green, (Santa Barbara, CA: ABC-CLIO, 2001), 298.

[184] International Taekwondo Federation, "Grand Master Trân Triêu Quân, MBA," January 6, 2015, https://www.taekwondoitf.org/tran-trieu-quan/.

[185] Gillis, Alex, A Killing Art: The Untold History of Tae Kwon Do, (United States: ECW Press, 2016), 82.

[186] Sánchez, García Raúl and Dale C. Spencer, *Fighting Scholars: Habitus and Ethnographies of Martial Arts and Combat Sports*, (London: Anthem Press, 2014), 176.

[187] Green, Thomas A., *Martial Arts of the World: An Encyclopedia*, (Santa Barbara, CA: ABC-CLIO, 2001).

[188] Goscha, Christopher E., *The Penguin History of Modern Vietnam*, (London: Penguin Books 2017), 479.

[189] Dan Hiergesell, "UFC: Paying Tribute to One of the World's Fastest Growing Sports." Bleacher Report, September 25, 2017, https://bleacherreport.com/articles/941301-ufc-paying-tribute-to-one-of-the-worlds-fastest-growing-sports.

[190] Roe, Augustus John, "An Investigation into the Effectiveness and Relevance of Traditional Vietnamese Martial Arts," Masters Thesis. Horizons University Paris, 2019.

CHAPTER FIVE FIGURES

Figure 30.—Nguyễn Trần Quang, Personal Collection—Bai Danh Chien 2, December 18 2018.

Conclusion

THE

FUTURE

OF

VIETNAMESE

MARTIAL

ARTS

CONCLUSION

Vietnam is truly a country with one foot in the future and one foot in the past. The nation is modernizing at a tremendous pace, yet despite these successes, the cultural roots of Vietnam still remain strong, fortified by its religious, historical and of course, martial arts practices.

At the time of writing this book, it is safe to say that the martial arts considered to be of Vietnamese origin still hold a strong connection with the Vietnamese people and for many, invoke a sense of nostalgia for days gone by.

Although there is an ever-growing presence of modern combat sports and self-defense systems, Vietnamese martial arts continue to be pursued by a critical mass of students, either as a casual pastime or a professional vocation. For now at least, it remains common to walk down the street of a Vietnamese city at the break of dawn and see the elderly practicing forms of *Thái Cực Quyền* (Tai Chi) or teenagers crammed into tiny martial arts gyms whose floors are stained with the blood, sweat and tears shed by the generations of disciples that came before them. While recent research has highlighted the divisions of opinion on the effectiveness of traditional Vietnamese martial arts, they are widely considered to be important cultural, historical and social practices that offer a range of benefits, both mental and physical.[191]

In this current climate, local systems of martial arts are more accessible to outsiders than they ever have been before. However, as the world becomes more united and globalized, the traditional martial arts of Vietnam (and indeed every nation) are at risk of eventually becoming homogenized or even lost entirely.

From my perspective on the ground in Vietnam, it appears likely that within a number of years the traditional martial arts forms of the country will be amalgamated into a uniform, nationalized system like those of Japanese *Budo* or Chinese *Wushu*. While this may be seen as a positive step toward modernization by some, traditionalists may disagree on the benefits of doing so. Therefore, this book hopes to preserve some aspects of traditional Vietnamese martial arts as they are found today.

Since I first arrived in Vietnam and began my study of Vietnamese martial arts, culture and language, I have traveled extensively throughout the country, meeting people from all backgrounds and walks of life. In doing so, I have been honored by the way that, as an outsider, I have been accepted into schools, communities and homes of the Vietnamese people and had the opportunity to experience some unique and amazing situations.

As a student, instructor, researcher of martial arts and traveler, I would urge any readers who may be interested, to visit the country, talk to the people, learn the language and participate in local martial arts. Following this page is a list of schools, throughout my research I have visited or met with students and masters from each of these institutions and I would wholeheartedly recommend every one of them. Regardless of age, race, language or ability you will always be warmly welcomed and there is no better time to do so than now.

Finally, I hope you have enjoyed reading "The Martial Arts of Vietnam" and I would love to hear your own stories or questions. Please contact me via "www.augustusjohnroe.com" or via social media and I will do my best to get back to you soon.

Augustus John Roe

Conclusion Notes

174 Roe, Augustus John, "An Investigation into the Effectiveness and Relevance of Traditional Vietnamese Martial Arts." Masters Thesis. Horizons University Paris, 2019

SCHOOLS/STYLES LISTING

Võ Phái Nhất Nam: Viet-Xo Friendship Palace, 79 Tran Hung Dao Street, Hai Ba Trung District, Hanoi.

Đấu Vật: Lieu Doi Village, Thanh Liem Hamlet, Ha Nam Province.

Võ Phái Nam Hồng Sơn: Quan Ngua Stadium, Ba Dinh District, Hanoi.

Vovinam: 221 Ly Thuong Kiet, Ward 15, District 11, Ho Chi Minh City.

Võ Đường Thanh Phong: Dong Xuan Ward, Hoan Kiem District, Hanoi.

Võ Cổ Truyền/Võ Tây Sơn: 09 Thanh Thai, Ward 14, District 10, Ho Chi Minh City.

Võ Đường Lý Tường: Dap Da District, An Nhon Hamlet, Binh Dinh Province.

Võ Đường Chùa Long Phước: Phuoc Thuan Village, Tuy Phuoc District, Binh Dinh Province.

Võ Đường Phi Long Vịnh: Phuoc Son Village, Tuy Phuoc District, Binh Dinh Province.

Vạn An Phái: Vo Kinh Van An School, Minh Mang Street, Hue, Hue Province.

Võ Đường Tinh Võ Đao: 129 Lam Van Ben Street, District 7, Ho Chi Minh City.

Võ Đường Bà Trà Tân Khánh/Takahado: Youth Culture House, No. 4, Pham Ngoc Thach Street, Ben Nghe Ward, District 1, Ho Chi Minh City.

Võ Đường Bình Định–Sa Long Cương: 4A, Pham Ngoc Thach Street, Ben Nghe Ward, District 1, Ho Chi Minh City.

That Son Than Quyen: Practiced throughout An Giang Province, Southwest Vietnam.

Bac Viet Vo: K30, Nguyen Hue Street, Lao Cai City, Lao Cai Province.

Quán Khí Đạo: Organization headquarters located outside of Vietnam.

Vịnh Xuân Quyền: Nguyen Tri Phuong University, 190 Quan Thanh Street, Ba Dinh District, Hanoi.

Nam Huyen Dao: Nam Chon Pagoda, 29 Tran Quang Khai, Tan Dinh Ward, District 1, Ho Chi Minh City.

Jeet Kune Do: 61 E Doc Vien Nhi Trung Uong, De La Thanh Street, Dong Da District, Hanoi.

Hung Gar Kung Fu: 04 Le Dai Hanh Street, Ward 15, District 11, Ho Chi Minh City.

Wushu/Sanda: 14, Trinh Hoai Duc Street, Ba Dinh District, Hanoi.

Karate: 36 Tran Phu Street, Ba Dinh District, Hanoi.

Aikido: Cau Giay Primary School, Lane 118, Nguyen Khanh Toan Street, Hanoi.

Kendo: Amsterdam High School Gymnasium, 01 Hoang Minh Giam Street, Cau Giay District, Hanoi.

Judo: Vietnam Judo Association, 36 Tran Phu Street, Ba Dinh District, Hanoi.

Taekwondo (WT): Vietnam Taekwondo Federation 4, Le Dai Hanh Street, Ho Chi Minh City.

Taekwondo (ITF): 15–17, 715 Ta Quang Buu Street, Ward 4, District 8, Ho Chi Minh City.

Escrima/Arnis: AKC Fitness, 6 Nguyen Truong To, Ba Dinh District, Hanoi

Muay Thai: Viet Muay Thai, 39 Bo De Street, Long Bien District, Hanoi.

Pencak Silat: Quan Ngua Stadium, Ba Dinh District Hanoi

Brazilian Jiu Jitsu: Ronin BJJ, CT1, Skylight Tower, Ngo Hoa Binh 6, Minh Khai, Hai Ba Trung District, Hanoi

Boxing: AKC Fitness, 6 Nguyen Truong To, Ba Dinh District, Hanoi

GLOSSARY

Annam (An Nam)—French protectorate of central Vietnam (1883–1948).

Áo Dài—Vietnamese traditional dress.

Âu Lạc—The early name of Vietnam (2879–258 BCE).

Bà—Old woman/grandma.

Bài Quyền—A martial arts form or kata.

Bảy—Seven

Bình Định—Province name simiar to the word "pacified" or "subjugated".

Cao Đài—A modern religion prevalent in south Vietnam, stemming from Tay Ninh Province.

Chăm—An ethnic minority people primarily in southwest Vietnam.

Champa—The former kingdom of the Cham people, which was dominant in central Vietnam between the seventh and seventeenth centuries.

Chợ—Market.

Chi Sao—(Chinese term) A pair drill commonly practiced in Vinh Xuan (Wing Chun).

Chùa—Pagoda.

Cổ Loa—The capital city of Au Lac.

Cochinchina (Nam Kỳ)—French colony of Southern Vietnam (1885–1945).

Chữ Nôm—The logographic script formerly used to write the Vietnamese language.

Cương-Nhu/Âm Dương—Hard-Soft/Yin-Yang.

Đại Việt—The former name of Vietnam from 1054–1400 CE, and again from 1428–1804 CE.

Đạo—Way/Path/Method (Chinese Tao/Japanese Do).

Đông Sơn—The Bronze Age culture in Vietnam.

Form—(English term) A set sequence of attacking and defensive movements.

Gia Định/Sài Gòn—The former names of Ho Chi Minh City. **Hmong**—An ethnic group prevalent in the mountains of Vietnam, Laos, China and Thailand.

Hồ Chí Minh—The revolutionary leader of Vietnam (May 19th, 1890 to September 2nd, 1969).

Hồ Dynasty—The Dynasty that ruled Vietnam from 1400–1406 CE.

Hòa Hảo (Sect)—A Buddhist group based in the Mekong Delta.

Huế—The former capital of Vietnam during the Nguyen Dynasty.

Khmer Krom—Vietnamese-Khmer.

(Early) Lê Dynasty—The Dynasty that ruled Vietnam between 980–1009 CE.

(Late) Lê Dynasty—The Dynasty that ruled Vietnam between 1428–1788 CE.

Lớn—Large/Big.

Lý Dynasty—The Dynasty that ruled Vietnam between 1009–1225 CE.

Nam Việt—The former name for modern day northern Vietnam from the Chinese   Nan Yue/南越.

Nguyễn Ánh/Gia Long—The first king of the Nguyen Dynasty.

Nguyễn Dynasty—The Dynasty that ruled Vietnam between 1802–1945 CE.

Nguyễn Huệ/Quang Trung—The first king to unite modern day Vietnam under unified rule/Tây Sơn rebellion leader.

Nguyễn Lữ—Younger brother of Nguyen Hue.

Nguyễn Nhạc—Older brother of Nguyen Hue.

Phong Thuỷ—Geomancy (Feng Shui/風水).

Quốc Ngữ—The 'modern' Latin script used for writing the Vietnamese language.

Sơn / Núi—Mountain.

Tây—West.

Tây Sơn District—The district where the three brothers Nguyen Hue, Nguyen

Lu and Nguyen Nhac came from and the focal point of the Tay Son Rebellion.

Tây Sơn Dynasty—The Dynasty that began from the Tay Son Rebellion.

Thăng Long—The former name of Hanoi, meaning "Soaring Dragon".

Tonkin (Bắc Kỳ) —French protectorate of northern Vietnam (1883–1948).

Trần Hưng Đạo/Trần Quốc Tuấn—The former King who repelled three Mongol invasions in the thirteenth century.

Trần Dynasty—The Dynasty that ruled Vietnam between 1225–1400 CE.

Trịnh—Feudal lords who controlled various provinces of Vietnam beween 1545–1787 CE.

Việt Minh—The northern Vietnamese communist army (the People's Army of Vietnam).

Võ—Fighting.

Võ Cổ Truyền—Traditional martial arts.

Võ Đường—Martial arts school.

Võ Hét—Traditional martial arts style (literally "Screaming Martial Arts").

Võ Phái—"Martial way".

Võ Tây Sơn—Martial arts of the Tay Son region.

Võ Thuật—Martial arts.

Qi (Chi)—(Chinese term) the circulating life force that serves as the basis for much of Chinese philosophy and traditional medicine.

Qigong—(Chinese term) the training of one's Qi through practices of breathing and physical movements.

Quyền—Form/fist.

ACKNOWLEDGMENTS

For their assistance in the writing, research, and photography of this book I would like to thank: Master Thich Quang Huyen of the Dharma Mountain Lineage, Master Tran Ha Manh of Nhat Nam Hanoi, Master Truong Van Vinh of the Phi Long Vinh School, Master Ho Tuong of the Ba Tra Tan Khanh School, Truong, Linh and Thuy of Lieu Doi Village, Master Hoang Thanh Phong of the Thanh Phong School, Dang Lai of the Bac Viet Vo School, Master Dinh Trong Thuy of the Vinh Xuan Kung Fu Viet Nam School, Viet Muay Thai Hanoi, Master Nguyen Thanh Bao of the Sa Long Cuong Ho Chi Minh City School, The District One Nam Huynh Dao School, Le Thai Duong of Brothers Judo School and Le Trung Linh of the Nam Hong Son Hanoi School.

I would like to thank: Le Thanh Ha for designing the layout and concept of the book, Ann Roe for her multiple proofreads and edits and, Dr Christopher Ford, Gaius Sision, Grant J. Riley, James Clarke, Jasper Roe, Jonathan Chappell and Joseph Williams for their assistance with photography, proofreading and editing.

ABOUT THE AUTHOR

Augustus John Roe is an author, linguist and instructor of traditional Vietnamese martial arts.

For more than a decade, he has lived and trained in Asia. During this time Augustus has worked on numerous television shows, books, magazines and academic projects documenting local cultures and martial arts practices.

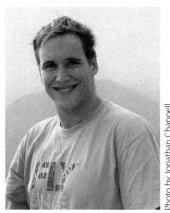

Photo by Jonathan Chappell

Augustus has a passion for language; he writes fiction, nonfiction and works as a freelance editor. His academic achievements include a Masters Degree in Martial Arts Studies and a Cambridge Delta qualification in language teaching.

Alongside traditional Vietnamese martial arts, Augustus had trained in Taekwondo, Wing Chun, iu Jitsu, Arnis, Muay Thai, Boxing, White Crane Kung Fu and more. He currently lives with his wife and children in Vietnam's capital city, Hanoi.

For more information about any of his writing or to contact Augustus, please visit www. augustusjohnroe.com or follow him on social media.

BOOKS FROM YMAA

101 REFLECTIONS ON TAI CHI CHUAN
108 INSIGHTS INTO TAI CHI CHUAN
A SUDDEN DAWN: THE EPIC JOURNEY OF BODHIDHARMA
A WOMAN'S QIGONG GUIDE
ADVANCING IN TAE KWON DO
ANALYSIS OF SHAOLIN CHIN NA 2ND ED
ANCIENT CHINESE WEAPONS
THE ART AND SCIENCE OF STAFF FIGHTING
THE ART AND SCIENCE OF STICK FIGHTING
ART OF HOJO UNDO
ARTHRITIS RELIEF, 3D ED.
BACK PAIN RELIEF, 2ND ED.
BAGUAZHANG, 2ND. ED.
BRAIN FITNESS
CARDIO KICKBOXING ELITE
CHIN NA IN GROUND FIGHTING
CHINESE FAST WRESTLING
CHINESE FITNESS
CHINESE TUI NA MASSAGE
CHOJUN
COMPLETE MARTIAL ARTIST
COMPREHENSIVE APPLICATIONS OF SHAOLIN CHIN NA
CONFLICT COMMUNICATION
CUTTING SEASON: A XENON PEARL MARTIAL ARTS THRILLER
DAO DE JING
DAO IN ACTION
DEFENSIVE TACTICS
DESHI: A CONNOR BURKE MARTIAL ARTS THRILLER
DIRTY GROUND
DR. WU'S HEAD MASSAGE
DUKKHA HUNGRY GHOSTS
DUKKHA REVERB
DUKKHA, THE SUFFERING: AN EYE FOR AN EYE
DUKKHA UNLOADED
ENZAN: THE FAR MOUNTAIN, A CONNOR BURKE MARTIAL ARTS
    THRILLER
ESSENCE OF SHAOLIN WHITE CRANE
EVEN IF IT KILLS ME
EXPLORING TAI CHI
FACING VIOLENCE
FIGHT BACK
FIGHT LIKE A PHYSICIST
THE FIGHTER'S BODY
FIGHTER'S FACT BOOK
FIGHTER'S FACT BOOK 2
THE FIGHTING ARTS
FIGHTING THE PAIN RESISTANT ATTACKER
FIRST DEFENSE
FORCE DECISIONS: A CITIZENS GUIDE
FOX BORROWS THE TIGER'S AWE
INSIDE TAI CHI
THE JUDO ADVANTAGE
THE JUJI GATAME ENCYCLOPEDIA
KAGE: THE SHADOW, A CONNOR BURKE MARTIAL ARTS
    THRILLER
KARATE SCIENCE
KATA AND THE TRANSMISSION OF KNOWLEDGE
KRAV MAGA COMBATIVES
KRAV MAGA PROFESSIONAL TACTICS
KRAV MAGA WEAPON DEFENSES
LITTLE BLACK BOOK OF VIOLENCE
LIUHEBAFA FIVE CHARACTER SECRETS
MARTIAL ARTS ATHLETE
MARTIAL ARTS INSTRUCTION
MARTIAL WAY AND ITS VIRTUES
MASK OF THE KING
MEDITATIONS ON VIOLENCE
MERIDIAN QIGONG EXERCISES
MIND/BODY FITNESS
MINDFUL EXERCISE
THE MIND INSIDE TAI CHI
THE MIND INSIDE YANG STYLE TAI CHI CHUAN
NATURAL HEALING WITH QIGONG
NORTHERN SHAOLIN SWORD, 2ND ED.
OKINAWA'S COMPLETE KARATE SYSTEM: ISSHIN RYU

THE PAIN-FREE BACK
PAIN-FREE JOINTS
POWER BODY
PRINCIPLES OF TRADITIONAL CHINESE MEDICINE
THE PROTECTOR ETHIC
QIGONG FOR HEALTH & MARTIAL ARTS 2ND ED.
QIGONG FOR LIVING
QIGONG FOR TREATING COMMON AILMENTS
QIGONG MASSAGE
QIGONG MEDITATION: EMBRYONIC BREATHING
QIGONG MEDITATION: SMALL CIRCULATION
QIGONG, THE SECRET OF YOUTH: DA MO'S CLASSICS
QUIET TEACHER: A XENON PEARL MARTIAL ARTS THRILLER
RAVEN'S WARRIOR
REDEMPTION
ROOT OF CHINESE QIGONG, 2ND ED.
SAMBO ENCYCLOPEDIA
SCALING FORCE
SELF-DEFENSE FOR WOMEN
SENSEI: A CONNOR BURKE MARTIAL ARTS THRILLER
SHIHAN TE: THE BUNKAI OF KATA
SHIN GI TAI: KARATE TRAINING FOR BODY, MIND, AND SPIRIT
SIMPLE CHINESE MEDICINE
SIMPLE QIGONG EXERCISES FOR HEALTH, 3RD ED.
SIMPLIFIED TAI CHI CHUAN, 2ND ED.
SOLO TRAINING
SOLO TRAINING 2
SPOTTING DANGER BEFORE IT SPOTS YOU
SUMO FOR MIXED MARTIAL ARTS
SUNRISE TAI CHI
SURVIVING ARMED ASSAULTS
TAE KWON DO: THE KOREAN MARTIAL ART
TAEKWONDO BLACK BELT POOMSAE
TAEKWONDO: A PATH TO EXCELLENCE
TAEKWONDO: ANCIENT WISDOM FOR THE MODERN WARRIOR
TAEKWONDO: DEFENSE AGAINST WEAPONS
TAEKWONDO: SPIRIT AND PRACTICE
TAI CHI BALL QIGONG: FOR HEALTH AND MARTIAL ARTS
TAI CHI BALL WORKOUT FOR BEGINNERS
THE TAI CHI BOOK
TAI CHI CHIN NA: THE SEIZING ART OF TAI CHI CHUAN,
    2ND ED.
TAI CHI CHUAN CLASSICAL YANG STYLE, 2ND ED.
TAI CHI CHUAN MARTIAL POWER, 3RD ED.
TAI CHI CONNECTIONS
TAI CHI DYNAMICS
TAI CHI FOR DEPRESSION
TAI CHI IN 10 WEEKS
TAI CHI QIGONG, 3RD ED.
TAI CHI SECRETS OF THE ANCIENT MASTERS
TAI CHI SECRETS OF THE WU & LI STYLES
TAI CHI SECRETS OF THE WU STYLE
TAI CHI SECRETS OF THE YANG STYLE
TAI CHI SWORD: CLASSICAL YANG STYLE, 2ND ED.
TAI CHI SWORD FOR BEGINNERS
TAI CHI WALKING
TAIJIQUAN THEORY OF DR. YANG, JWING-MING
TAO OF BIOENERGETICS
TENGU: THE MOUNTAIN GOBLIN, A CONNOR BURKE MARTIAL
    ARTS THRILLER
TIMING IN THE FIGHTING ARTS
TRADITIONAL CHINESE HEALTH SECRETS
TRADITIONAL TAEKWONDO
TRAINING FOR SUDDEN VIOLENCE
TRUE WELLNESS
TRUE WELLNESS: THE MIND
TRUE WELLNESS FOR YOUR HEART
THE WARRIOR'S MANIFESTO
WAY OF KATA
WAY OF SANCHIN KATA
WAY TO BLACK BELT
WESTERN HERBS FOR MARTIAL ARTISTS
WILD GOOSE QIGONG
WINNING FIGHTS
WISDOM'S WAY

DVDS FROM YMAA

ADVANCED PRACTICAL CHIN NA IN-DEPTH
ANALYSIS OF SHAOLIN CHIN NA
ATTACK THE ATTACK
BAGUA FOR BEGINNERS 1
BAGUA FOR BEGINNERS 2
BAGUAZHANG: EMEI BAGUAZHANG
BEGINNER QIGONG FOR WOMEN 1
BEGINNER QIGONG FOR WOMEN 2
BEGINNER TAI CHI FOR HEALTH
CHEN STYLE TAIJIQUAN
CHEN TAI CHI FOR BEGINNERS
CHIN NA IN-DEPTH COURSES 1—4
CHIN NA IN-DEPTH COURSES 5—8
CHIN NA IN-DEPTH COURSES 9—12
FACING VIOLENCE: 7 THINGS A MARTIAL ARTIST MUST KNOW
FIVE ANIMAL SPORTS
FIVE ELEMENTS ENERGY BALANCE
INFIGHTING
INTRODUCTION TO QI GONG FOR BEGINNERS
JOINT LOCKS
KNIFE DEFENSE: TRADITIONAL TECHNIQUES AGAINST A DAGGER
KUNG FU BODY CONDITIONING 1
KUNG FU BODY CONDITIONING 2
KUNG FU FOR KIDS
KUNG FU FOR TEENS
LOGIC OF VIOLENCE
MERIDIAN QIGONG
NEIGONG FOR MARTIAL ARTS
NORTHERN SHAOLIN SWORD : SAN CAI JIAN, KUN WU JIAN, QI MEN JIAN
QI GONG 30-DAY CHALLENGE
QI GONG FOR ANXIETY
QI GONG FOR ARMS, WRISTS, AND HANDS
QIGONG FOR BEGINNERS: FRAGRANCE
QI GONG FOR BETTER BREATHING
QI GONG FOR CANCER
QI GONG FOR ENERGY AND VITALITY
QI GONG FOR HEADACHES
QI GONG FOR HEALING
QI GONG FOR HEALTHY JOINTS
QI GONG FOR HIGH BLOOD PRESSURE
QIGONG FOR LONGEVITY
QI GONG FOR STRONG BONES
QI GONG FOR THE UPPER BACK AND NECK
QIGONG FOR WOMEN
QIGONG FOR WOMEN WITH DAISY LEE
QIGONG MASSAGE
QIGONG MINDFULNESS IN MOTION
QIGONG: 15 MINUTES TO HEALTH
SABER FUNDAMENTAL TRAINING
SAI TRAINING AND SEQUENCES
SANCHIN KATA: TRADITIONAL TRAINING FOR KARATE POWER
SCALING FORCE
SHAOLIN KUNG FU FUNDAMENTAL TRAINING: COURSES 1 & 2
SHAOLIN LONG FIST KUNG FU: ADVANCED SEQUENCES 1
SHAOLIN LONG FIST KUNG FU: ADVANCED SEQUENCES 2
SHAOLIN LONG FIST KUNG FU: BASIC SEQUENCES
SHAOLIN LONG FIST KUNG FU: INTERMEDIATE SEQUENCES
SHAOLIN SABER: BASIC SEQUENCES
SHAOLIN STAFF: BASIC SEQUENCES
SHAOLIN WHITE CRANE GONG FU BASIC TRAINING: COURSES 1 & 2

SHAOLIN WHITE CRANE GONG FU BASIC TRAINING: COURSES 3 & 4
SHUAI JIAO: KUNG FU WRESTLING
SIMPLE QIGONG EXERCISES FOR HEALTH
SIMPLE QIGONG EXERCISES FOR ARTHRITIS RELIEF
SIMPLE QIGONG EXERCISES FOR BACK PAIN RELIEF
SIMPLIFIED TAI CHI CHUAN: 24 & 48 POSTURES
SIMPLIFIED TAI CHI FOR BEGINNERS 48
SUNRISE TAI CHI
SUNSET TAI CHI
SWORD: FUNDAMENTAL TRAINING
TAEKWONDO KORYO POOMSAE
TAI CHI BALL QIGONG: COURSES 1 & 2
TAI CHI BALL QIGONG: COURSES 3 & 4
TAI CHI BALL WORKOUT FOR BEGINNERS
TAI CHI CHUAN CLASSICAL YANG STYLE
TAI CHI CONNECTIONS
TAI CHI ENERGY PATTERNS
TAI CHI FIGHTING SET
TAI CHI FIT: 24 FORM
TAI CHI FIT: FLOW
TAI CHI FIT: FUSION BAMBOO
TAI CHI FIT: FUSION FIRE
TAI CHI FIT: FUSION IRON
TAI CHI FIT: HEART HEALTH WORKOUT
TAI CHI FIT IN PARADISE
TAI CHI FIT: OVER 50
TAI CHI FIT OVER 50: BALANCE EXERCISES
TAI CHI FIT OVER 50: SEATED WORKOUT
TAI CHI FIT OVER 60: GENTLE EXERCISES
TAI CHI FIT OVER 60: HEALTHY JOINTS
TAI CHI FIT OVER 60: LIVE LONGER
TAI CHI FIT: STRENGTH
TAI CHI FIT: TO GO
TAI CHI FOR WOMEN
TAI CHI FUSION: FIRE
TAI CHI QIGONG
TAI CHI PUSHING HANDS: COURSES 1 & 2
TAI CHI PUSHING HANDS: COURSES 3 & 4
TAI CHI SWORD: CLASSICAL YANG STYLE
TAI CHI SWORD FOR BEGINNERS
TAI CHI SYMBOL: YIN YANG STICKING HANDS
TAIJI & SHAOLIN STAFF: FUNDAMENTAL TRAINING
TAIJI CHIN NA IN-DEPTH
TAIJI 37 POSTURES MARTIAL APPLICATIONS
TAIJI SABER CLASSICAL YANG STYLE
TAIJI WRESTLING
TRAINING FOR SUDDEN VIOLENCE
UNDERSTANDING QIGONG 1: WHAT IS QI? • HUMAN QI CIRCULATORY SYSTEM
UNDERSTANDING QIGONG 2: KEY POINTS • QIGONG BREATHING
UNDERSTANDING QIGONG 3: EMBRYONIC BREATHING
UNDERSTANDING QIGONG 4: FOUR SEASONS QIGONG
UNDERSTANDING QIGONG 5: SMALL CIRCULATION
UNDERSTANDING QIGONG 6: MARTIAL QIGONG BREATHING
WATER STYLE FOR BEGINNERS
WHITE CRANE HARD & SOFT QIGONG
YANG TAI CHI FOR BEGINNERSS
WUDANG KUNG FU: FUNDAMENTAL TRAINING
WUDANG SWORD
WUDANG TAIJIQUAN
XINGYIQUAN

more products available from . . .
YMAA Publication Center, Inc. 楊氏東方文化出版中心
1-800-669-8892 • info@ymaa.com • www.ymaa.com

YMAA
PUBLICATION CENTER

CPSIA information can be obtained
at www.ICGtesting.com
Printed in the USA
JSHW011158160820
7254JS00006B/17